AF333381

A FRESH LOOK
AT
HANSEN'S DISEASE

A FRESH LOOK
AT
HANSEN'S DISEASE

M. J. de Mallac

VANTAGE PRESS
New York

FIRST EDITION
All rights reserved, including the right of
reproduction in whole or in part in any form.

Copyright © 1992 by M. J. de Mallac

Published by Vantage Press, Inc.
516 West 34th Street, New York, New York 10001

Manufactured in the United States of America
ISBN: 0-533-09237-X

Library of Congress Catalog Card No.: 90-90267

0 9 8 7 6 5 4 3 2 1

This monograph is humbly dedicated to all those patients who, in the name of "leprosy," are eluding detection from fear of being recognized, left in the lurch, excluded from work, refused medical care, denied hospitalization, abandoned by their folk, or shunned by the community still.

"Don't think, look!" advocated Ludwig Wittgenstein (1889–1951). Since one has been so far looking at Hansen's disease and the patient mostly from the outside, it is high time to look at the disease, and moreso, the patient, from the inside too.

Facts, according to Marcel Proust (1871–1922), do not penetrate the world of our beliefs: they haven't triggered them off nor can they destroy them. One may add that the emphasis lies equally on the implications and consequences of those facts.

Adding, to be sure, further weight to the evidence, yet upon the injunction of William the Silent (1533–1584), that it is not necessary to hope in order to understand, nor necessary to succeed in order to persevere.

Contents

Acknowledgment   xi

The Gist of It All   1
The Age-Old Legacy   7
The Immunological Dispensation   49
The Crux of the Matter   69
The Essential Reality of the Disease   103
The Channels of Control   122
Summing Up   150

General Bibliography   155
Author Index   159

Acknowledgment

The present writer wishes to express his gratitude to: Professor A. Rotberg of Brazil for having provided a great deal of the material needed for the etymological and social considerations under the "Punitive Label," all of it for the elaboration of the "Saga of the Name Change," and the World Health Organization, Geneva, for permission to quote at length some of Professor B. R. Bloom's remarks in "Towards a Leprosy Vaccine," *World Health,* May 1985.

A FRESH LOOK
AT
HANSEN'S DISEASE

The Gist of It All

The reality of Hansen's disease[1] displaying complexities of a somewhat bewildering nature, one is left with a vision of the disease precisely to the extent that it should not be confused with that reality.[2]

Each era is laden with its toll of epidemics or plagues which, part of the ecosystem, have changed the course of human events as has been reported. Hence, Black Death in the Middle Ages,[3] the upsurge of syphilis during the Renaissance,[4] smallpox at the time of the conquest of the New World, tuberculosis along the Romantic Period,[5] and the 1918 influenza wild spree.[6] While the daunting magnitude of AIDS dominates the contemporary scene, Hansen's disease remains committed to its archetypal grip of quite a different order.

What of a "chronic granulomatous response to persistent non-viable mycobacterial antigens, the complex of possible non-specific findings,"[7] revealed for the first time to the scientific world in 1847 with the publication of Danielssen and Boeck's "Om Spedalsked"? What of this most complex of all mycobacterial diseases not confined to our species anymore? Why the attraction for a disease apart that "occupies a long-awaited seat among essential health priorities, when biomedical research in various fields of the disease has remained far behind that of most other diseases?" (Bloom, 1985)

Well Hansen's disease is not just another communicable disease, as erroneously postulated in some quarters. Its significance is brought about by the evidence that, in spite of a relatively low prevalence of the disease,

- There are but few other afflictions known to man that stretch back with equal historicity. None that practically in every culture has evoked—and still does—deep-rooted aversion and fear, linked in part to the isolation of the patients practised in the past

(McDougall & Yamalkar, 1987), hence enticing patients to conceal the nature of their illness from all but close relatives and friends in order to avoid social ostracism (Rolston & Chesteen, 1970).

- The disease is "one of several conditions which the majority of people place in a category apart—and place apart is what they do their best to achieve,"[8] hence the numerous ramifications of Hansen's disease governing traditional belief systems among lay public and the patients themselves.
- The disease is imbued with "a rich and complex mythology, and in Western cultures is perhaps unsurpassed in its ability to evoke adverse social responses" (Neylan et al., 1986).
- There is no other illness with such psychological impact on both the patient and his community, none whatever with so much stigma.
- The disease is "unique in the immuno-pathologic complex that gives it its identity" (Skinsnes, 1964), hence the diversity and variety in its manifestations.[9]
- The causative organism—able to persist for months or years following effective chemotherapy—has still not been shown to fulfill Koch's postulate.[10] With a generation time[11] exceeding by far that of any known bacterium, it is the only one of its species to invade peripheral nerves.
- The mode of transmission of that least communicable of diseases—probably as a consequence of the long latency or incubation period—is unknown still.
- Hansen's disease is the major cause of peripheral neuropathy, the third leading cause of blindness worldwide,[12] hence the most widespread crippling disease to date as generally acknowledged.
- "Perhaps in no other disease are the results of early diagnosis so rich. Perhaps in no other disease are the penalties of neglect so terrible."[13]

However deeply ingrained in collective memory, language, and culture, it is clear that, by now, Hansen's disease offers quite a wide range of challenges. Thus,

- to the epidemiologist, the disease spells a serious health problem[14] whereby control of the disease—geared over the past twenty-five years mainly to secondary prevention—has not come up to expectations, because of inappropriate detection of individuals at risk, and their protection through epidemiological intervention, i.e., primary prevention.

- To the microbiologist and some hansenologists (leprologists), the causative organism is the chief proponent, warranting further knowledge of its basic biology and its more dramatic elimination than is presently the case.
- To the pathologist, more fundamental insight into the nature of the immunopathological process of the disease is called for.
- To the immunologist, basic scientists, and other hansenologists (leprologists), the target is adequate immunodiagnostic and immunoprophylactic tools, as well as overcoming the selective immunological unresponsiveness in polar multibacillary (PM) or LL patients.
- To the social scientists (social psychologists, medical anthropologists, sociologists, historians), Hansen's disease is a new yet unique field of research in human behavior.
- To the social worker, the disease—as a socioeconomic problem of far-reaching magnitude and consequences—takes precedence over its clinical aspects.
- To the health care administrator, the task is how to achieve a realistic and cost-effective goal in controlling the disease.
- To the executive of a philanthropic organization or voluntary organization, the prime appeal is the haunting spectrum of deformities or mutilations.
- What it is that concerns the hansenologist (leprologist) most is a matter of personal outlook. It seems that viewing the disease as an integrated whole would be more to the point, yet without losing sight of the patient.

While, admittedly, Hansen's disease still posits a good deal of unanswered questions within the ambit of its epidemiological, microbiological, immunological, and clinico-pathological features, the disease is no more the poor relative of tropical medicine. Gone are "the contradictions, evasions and unscientific deductions that bestrew much of the literature on leprosy."[15]

Short, perhaps, on the part of the present writer to look at Hansen's disease with a beginner's mind,[16] he has chosen instead to "rethink" some of the traditional ideas and views of the disease process. Hence the grass-root nature of his approach that, incidentally, does not aim at the definitive, but builds towards certain specific yet limited areas. In this respect, reaching across accepted belief systems of that sort is bound to entail rebuttals, notwithstanding the unorthodox stand of the present writer for which, on both counts, he would be solely responsible.

As regards this monograph, and at variance with usual procedure, room is made at the onset for the hansenian (leprosy patient), i.e., his psychology, age-old legacy, the punitive label he shares in common with the disease so as to lend cogency, if not substance, to the alternate terminology used in the text and the advocacy of the name change expounded later on. In this connection, let it be made quite clear that the use of alternative terminology is neither a deliberate attempt nor a challenge, rather an exercise in feasibility which, borne out of exceptional circumstances, is equally left to the appreciation of the reader.

Irrespective of how Hansen's bacillus (*M. leprae*) gets into the body, what determines, and brings about, nerve and tissue involvement is the central issue that confers to the disease its fundamental immunological status: Hansen's disease, by virtue of its polymorphous and spectral nature, is a continuum reflecting at one end the polar paucibacillary (PP) or TT form as the outcome of cell-mediated immunity (CMI), at the other end polar multibacillary (PM) or LL form as an immuno-deficient complex, and with the borderline group at the center implying a shifting balance.

Peripheral neuropathy, as the primary reality of the disease, takes precedence over skin and other tissues as has hitherto not been the case in both clinical and didactic practice.

The possible sequence of events from incipient infection with Hansen's bacillus (*M. leprae*) to overt manifestation of the disease is laid down in a novel pre-clinical and clinical conceptual framework.

Control of the disease is not elaborated as such since it is more authoritatively dealt with elsewhere. Rather the various channels of that control are critically appraised, equally in keeping with the experience of the present writer in the field.

The summing up, couched in a more philosophical mood, reflects a personal credo concerning the main topics of the text, both of which presumably are not to the expectations of academically-oriented colleagues and past collaborators.

Wherever appropriate, significant comments of various authors are quoted at length in the text for the sole purpose of illustrating the point. Notes are meant to punctuate or enlarge on those terms or points wherever desirable, while at the same time enjoying an unmitigated freedom of expression.

Finally, given the seminal role of immunology in Hansen's disease, and while much has, indeed, been learnt in recent years, it is not made easier for the lay physician to penetrate into the arcane world of the immunologist, moreso when grappling with the complex jargon of the basic scientist.[17] Even though the gap between immunology and hansenology (leprology) is called upon to be filled, the present writer has adopted a less sophisticated language when it comes to relating these two disciplines, bearing in mind that, in the case of the former, its explosive growth requires constant updating,[18] while in the case of the latter it is a disease process given to the vagaries of change.

Notes

1. Term adopted throughout for reasons to be made explicit.
2. In other words, Hansen's disease is much more than meets the eye.
3. Or "bubonic" plague, which wiped out as much as a third of Europe's population.
4. The great wave of the disease spread over Europe in the sixteenth century.
5. Up to a point, though, since according to Lyall Watson, "There is a skeletal evidence of the effect of tuberculosis in graves from Germany dating back 10,000 years—and similar evidence from Old Kingdom in ancient Egypt." (in *Supernature II*, 1986)
6. A pandemic, the virulence of which for unknown reasons claimed a reported 20 million lives within a few months.
7. *The Lancet*, leading article, January 21, 1967.
8. A medical man, editorial, *Leprosy Review*, 1972. In this respect, Lichtwardt (1948) goes further: "No one disease has been so shamefully misunderstood, and so disgracefully misrepresented as that relatively non-contagious condition, which most of the world still knows as 'leprosy.'"
9. For instance, as has been asked, why does the overwhelming majority of the population at risk never develop the disease? Why does only a minority show immunological unresponsiveness to the antigens of Hansen's bacillus (*M. leprae*)?
10. I.e. it is the only organism that still defies cultivation on artificial media.
11. Time taken for the organism to double or divide into two by binary fission.
12. An estimated 750,000 to 1 million people.
13. Remark from the present writer (1967).
14. Populations at risk are said to exceed one billion. The patient population itself is between twelve and fifteen million worldwide, a third to a fourth of whom are

on regular treatment, a fifth to a fourth facing the threat of permanent and progressive disability and/or deformity.

15. *The Lancet*, leading article, January 27, 1968.
16. In keeping with what the late Dr. Frans Hemerijckx confided to the present writer over twenty-five years ago: "*Il faudrait repenser la lèpre!*" (One ought to rethink leprosy!) Or simply because "there is a certain ethos in one's culture that it is better to look at things without bias or preference. Look at them to the point of not going back."
17. Most basic scientists and some immunologists are partly responsible for this. To paraphrase Gary Zukav: "Their shop talk sounds like advanced Greek, unless you are Greek and one of them. When they are not talking to their peers, they speak English again. Ask them what they do, however, and they sound like the natives of Corfu again" (in *The Dancing Wu Li Masters*, 1979).
18. As J. Kaplan, National Jewish Centre for Immunology, puts it, "The field of immunology is progressing so rapidly that the journals are out of date by the time they are published."

References

A Medical Man. The Stigma of Leprosy—A Personal Experience. *Lep. Rev.* 43 (1972): 83–84.

Bloom. B.R. Towards a Leprosy Vaccine. *World Health*, May 1985, 3–5.

Lichtwardt, H.A. Why Not Change the Name? *The Star*, 1948.

McDougall, A.C.M. and Yamalkar, S.J. Leprosy. Basic Information and Management, CIBA-GEIGY, 1987.

Mallac (de), M.J. Onset and Pattern of Deformity in Leprosy. *Lep. Rev.* 37 (1967): 71–91.

Neylan, T.C. et al. Illness Beliefs of Leprosy Patients. Use of Medical Anthropology in Clinical Practice. *Int. J. Lep.* 56 (1988): 231–137.

Rolston, R.H. and Chesteen, H.E. The Identification of Psychological Factors Related to the Rehabilitation of Leprosy Patients. Final Report RD 2316-P, The School of Social Welfare, Louisiana State University, Baton Rouge, 1970.

The Age-Old Legacy

> "The essential tragedy of Hansen's disease is
> the tragedy of opportunities missed."[1]

The approach to a disease—moreso by virtue of the intricacies and/or complexities of that disease—stems, admittedly, from a personal outlook. In the case of Hansen's disease, an exception to the established rule is made here since it primarily embodies the coexistence of three factors: the disease, the patient, and the designation they share in common while traditionally associated with shame and disgrace.[2]

The Disease Apart

> "Hansen's disease claims a certain excep-
> tionalism, a special nature that derives from its
> time-honoured shunted uniqueness."

When writing about Hansen's disease,[3] it ought to be appreciated in the first place that it belongs to a much wider context than generally recognized. Thus,

- it is reported that the sheer disparity in the quality of life between the Third World—where, incidentally, three-quarters of the planet's population lives—and the more privileged countries, an already telling enough evidence, is furthermore shadowed by what diseases of greatest concern among underprivileged nations get: a mere pittance as compared to what the West spends on its national security. Besides, Bloom (1985) intimates that only 1–2% of the total global medical research is devoted to diseases from which two-thirds of the world population is suffering.

- As a disease of the sub-tropical and tropical areas, Hansen's disease is conceptually part of

  those diseases of poverty, in the sense that they are due to deficiencies and hazards and could be prevented if resources were unlimited (in extreme case, by removal of populations from hazardous areas). In practice, however, resources are severely restricted, and as the tropical diseases frequently do not respond to simple improvement in conditions of life, the solution must come from new knowledge obtained through laboratory, clinical, epidemiological and socioeconomic research.[4]

- In the poorest endemic countries, Hansen's disease stands out as one disease among other diseases, one public health problem among other public health problems (Lechat, 1981), with far less dramatic impact in terms of numbers: schistosomiasis, onchocerciasis or river blindness, malaria,[5] tuberculosis, sleeping sickness, gastroenteritis,[6] malnutrition, and avitaminosis affecting hundreds of millions of human beings. As a result, little wonder that Hansen's disease is given low priority and, consequently, is not viewed in its true perspective, hence the lack of global strategy it warrants as equally pointed out by Lechat.

- Hansen's disease and the various attitudes it generates vary from one region to another, from one country to another within that region, presumably from one community to another within that country. Moreover, from one generation to the next. It follows that the disease is not prone to identical stigmatization the world over: it is a question of nature and degree within cultural and conceptual variations, as has been observed. By the same token, in endemic countries allowance is to be made as regards differences in both educational levels and awareness of the disease from a community viewpoint and social background, with communication between health care personnel and the patients coming into it, too.

  The magnitude of the problem relating to Hansen's disease worldwide can only be roughly estimated, not adequately assessed, owing to scarcity of information, mere statistical evidence, besides not reflecting the true extent of human plight involved.

- Knowledge of the disease is marred at the outset by the inability to single out those determinants that would explain (i) the latency or long incubation period of the disease, (ii) sub-clinical infection, (iii) the identification, development, pattern, and transmission of the disease, as has been remarked.

- Perhaps the most intriguing feature of Hansen's disease, as indicated by Ottenhoff and de Vries (1988), is the interindividual variability on clinical grounds appearing in the course of the disease. Perhaps the most encouraging element is that, according to Hastings (1985), "in many areas research is called upon to unravel the various pieces of the puzzle Hansen's disease presents."

- The lower the prevalence of Hansen's disease in a given area, the less alert public and professional awareness of the disease, the less degree of suspicion, even though the reverse is not necessarily so. Moreover, as expressed by many authors, the danger for the populations at risk stems more from the undiagnosed infectious patients than from those same patients on treatment.

- Despite laudable efforts and dedication from all quarters in the common fight against the disease, and encouraging results at all levels concerned, the other side of the picture is—more often than not—compounded of non-integrated control services, poor or non-existent notification, inadequate health care, overlooking of early diagnosis from medical and paramedical staff alike, and neglect and indifference of the patients themselves.

- An estimated twelve to fifteen million people are affected by Hansen's disease in the world today. Of these, only about half have been diagnosed and registered, and probably one-third to one-fourth of these registered patients are under regular treatment as reported by Noordeen (1988).

The historical background of the disease has been scholarly dealt with elsewhere.[7] Even though an ancient disease, though unlikely to be the oldest affliction known to man as generally believed, Hansen's disease was probably unknown in Biblical times, and did not make its appearance until the late pre-Christian era in Europe (Tas, 1953). No other disease has been ever since—and still is—prone to so many misconceptions, inaccuracies, and distortion bordering on the medieval, or to the extent that the disease is "engrossed by legendary reminiscences, inflated notions and unconscious sense of aversion" in the words of Letayf (1955).

In his enquiry in south China about the concepts associated with Hansen's disease, Skinsnes (1964) reports that in this region:

> Leprosy has been regarded as a punishment from heaven for moral misdemeanor. . . . Persons who contracted leprosy are thought to be transgressors of moral law and likely to be morally suspect. . . . Leprosy has been regarded as a venereal disease. . . . Bodily discharges, body heat, skin scrapings, etc. from persons with leprosy have been regarded as noxious elements, and since persons having the disease are believed to be evil, they have often been suspected of using those elements to harm society. . . . The gods can cure all diseases except leprosy, and there is no hope for those with this infection. . . . Leprosy is thought to be hereditary for three generations and the children of parents with leprosy are considered certain to acquire the disease. . . . Leprosy patients may "sell" the disease to others and cure themselves through sexual contacts with varying number of healthy persons.

Languillon (1986) intimates, in turn, that the concept of the disease means equally moral guilt, sin, a group of cutaneous manifestations, among which Hansen's disease, all together known as the religious syndrome.[8]

Acknowledged as the legacy of the poor and the destitute in most instances, with its attendant overcrowding, promiscuity, malnutrition, unhygienic conditions, and illiteracy, Hansen's disease bears the brunt of opprobrium still, in that "no disease exists in society as a pure disease, but acts through the institutions, attitudes, and responses of that society" (Ell, 1987), or in spite of the fact that Hansen's disease "is not purely a medical affair, but an issue for us all" (Lechat, 1981). Browne (1981) enjoins more forcibly when he writes that:

> We live in a world where leprosy is not diagnosed early; where preventable deformity has not been—and is not being—prevented. In short, we live in a world inhabited by fellow human beings suffering from the disease called leprosy and also suffering from what they think, what other people think of them and their disease.

Hansen's disease entails multifaceted ramifications that, even after successful therapy, pervade the life of the patients. Despite social acceptance in some areas or improvement as to actual social reactions to the patients in other areas reported by Meisels-Navon (1988), there is according to the author "a gradual process of dissociation between leprosy as a social phenomenon and leprosy as a cultural metaphor which accompanies the medical achievements." In other words, the paradox of the disease is that its image is negatively perpetuated while the illness is attended to, or has been cured.

The Archetypal Outsider

> "Prior to the discovery of Hansen's bacillus, medicine was making its way through history by blundering off into oblivion the very existence of the leprosy patient."[9]

Some insight into the psychology of Hansen's disease is warranted, bearing in mind that such a subject, while occupying a modest place in the literature,[10] is a fairly recent one though enhanced by personal experience.

Some of the concepts associated with the disease have been discussed in the preceding section, yet in another vein it is clear that the "fear or terror surrounding the word leprosy comes from the idea of gross deformity and open sores," these furthermore "not directly attributable to the disease itself, but as a result of loss of sensation thus allowing the patient to deform himself" (Brand, 1981).

This view is hardly shared by, or known to, the members of the profession, practically not at all by the public at large and society in particular: for centuries the image of Hansen's disease has been—and still is—linked to the neglected or late stage of the disease.

As regards the hansenian himself (leprosy patient), any approach to his psychology would have to take into account his pre-existing personality, etho-cultural background, and socioeconomic status, the traditional or made-up representation of the disease, his community's attitude to his illness, the extent to which the patient is bound to, or influenced by, these interrelated existential factors. Besides, as remarked by Del Cerro (1968), attitudes and perceptions of the patient's family are important, too.

While Shanmuganandan et al. (1989) observe that "the psychological response of the leprosy patient in the long range depends upon personal significance and this is due mainly to the influence of the environment, attitude towards his illness, culture mores and societal norms," it is interesting to note that, in their investigation of the psychological world of the hansenian (leprosy patient) by means of the Minnesota Multiphasic Personality Inventory (MMPI), Flynn and Harvey (1968), correlating interview and questionnaire material, found no common Hansen's disease personality.

One way or another, more so when he is an educated one—the hansenian (leprosy patient) lives in a world that equates himself alone as has been pointed out, and in some countries like Brazil the patient is a "social being affected in his own integrity by a disease complex called leprosy" (Letayf, 1955).

If subject to physical handicap, the patient, in the words of Kaufmann et al. (1986), shows a feeling of insecurity and signs of regression through the tendency of depending on others as a means of relieving his problems. His body image is liable to be distorted through feeling himself diminished, inferior, ashamed, even unworthy of the respect of his surroundings. The response, still according to these authors, that the handicapped hansenians (leprosy patients) share in common is an overwhelming sense of loss.

The environment of the patient is apt from the start to make him feel different from other healthy individuals and, moreover, set apart from them as has been observed. Whether the hansenian (leprosy patient) is more affected by the sheer impact of his illness than by his community's attitude, or vice versa, is mutually inclusive: what is at stake is the patient's altered identity when moreso brought about by physical handicap.

At the psychological level, this is altogether a specific situation ranging from low self-respect to feeling of shame or disgust through presumably inherent or acquired guilt complex, loss of object, or a sense of fatalism or surrender as has been reported. To make it more explicit, it means the likelihood of anxiety neurosis, somatization of the patient's problems, depression, paranoid delusion, or suicidal ideation as has been put forth elsewhere.[11,12,13,14]

More dramatic is the occurrence of suicide per se as mentioned by Letayf (1955) in Brazil, so also the case in China as reported by Skinsnes (1964) as follows:

Suicide is contemplated by many and accepted as the final solution by not a few. Thus one villager related that ten years previously there lived in a village known to him a married woman having four sons. When she found that she contracted leprosy she wished to die and requested that her family bury her alive. They dug a hole in the ground, she jumped in, and so was interred as she requested. In Formosa, of a group of about two hundred young men with early leprosy, fifteen committed suicide within a period of a few months.

Zhou et al. (1988) say that social discrimination against hansenians (leprosy patients) in the People's Republic of China is one of the causes of suicide. For instance, the suicide rate among them in Baoing County, Jiangsu Province, was over 100 to 1 as compared with the suicide rate per hundred thousand in the general population.

Those familiar with field work conditions in Third World countries would hardly disagree that, more often than not, the average hansenian (leprosy patient) is not given the benefit of ready attention nor taken care of in good time nor educated to cope all along with the modalities of his illness. In endemic and partially endemic areas, a concerted awareness of the patient as a person[15] proves the exception (cf specialized institutions), a fragmented approach and therapeutic coverage the rule at rural levels: the likelihood for the patient to feel devalued is all there. Moreover, the chances are that—whether he reports for treatment early or late, recognizes or ignores the first signs of the disease—the hansenian (leprosy patient) is already a candidate for ostracism.[16]

It seems that enquiring whether the patient (i) matters first and foremost as a person, (ii) is offered the means to retrieve his integrity, (iii) his life yearns for something else, (iv) his sensitivities are safeguarded, or (v) his dignity is upheld as has been emphasized[17] would be relevant yet pointing to another direction: the hansenian (leprosy patient), as has also been said, is relinquished to inevitabilities. He is the archetypal outsider par excellence, i.e., edged away from his community, an extraterritorial to common humanity in keeping with the Levitical precept that, according to Fleming (1989), he should dwell "without the camp."[18] Much more than is presently the case with other communicable diseases the status of the hansenian (leprosy patient) is geared to utter sensitivity, even though exceptions do exist. More often than not, the patient foots the bill for something neither of his own making nor with which he has anything to do. In short, the patient—particularly in endemic areas—is granted no voice: he is submitted to the policy of the healthy majority as has been remarked, yet that very majority for whom it is easier to pass by and, while not necessarily dismissing the patient, avoid looking into his eyes, thereby shunning reality. Little wonder, then, that at the limit the average hansenian (leprosy patient), when branded and treated like dross, finds himself "in a world as if offended by his presence."[19]

More significantly in another respect, the psychology of a human being deprived of sensation in his limb(s) and/or face—as is presently the case with most hansenians (leprosy patients)—evokes a situation neither emphasized enough nor fathomed properly: the "mute skin" postulated by Lechat (1980) is probably the most disconcerting feature of the actual issue.

One is reminded by Bryceson (1981) that the body image of the normal person is based upon sensory input from his or her body and, consequently, when he or she loses sensation in a limb loses that limb from his or her conscious mind. In this respect, hansenians (leprosy patients) confided to Brand (1981) that they felt as though they were walking on blocks of wood, which have been fastened to the stumps of their legs. They might, furthermore, look upon their hands as tools or implements which, although dead, serve some purpose. Brand thinks that "in the subconscious mind of these patients they do not have hands and feet."

When it comes to the eyes of the patient, another author writes that:

> Blindness in the individual who has not lost normal skin sensitivity is enough of a handicap, but in one who has lost this faculty it is disastrous. Few have the resources, material, mental, and spiritual, to live with it.[20]

In other words, the hansenian (leprosy patient) affected by loss of sensation in his limb(s) and/or face has forgotten what feeling was like. He has no idea where hand(s), arm(s), foot/feet, or leg(s) are if he could not see them, none whether his affected face is smiling or in a deep frown. His overall impression remains as if his extremity(ies) had become absent or dead to themselves. He is deprived—moreover—and never to be given back—of that alarm system, that protective mechanism to safeguard the integrity of his body: pain.

Whether what has been commented upon so far measures up with one's sense of awareness or not, the evidence is that somewhere along the line something else in our dealings with the hansenian (leprosy patient) went amiss, was overlooked or neglected. Perhaps it has not been understood that contracting Hansen's is not just being affected by another communicable disease, but an illness that, far more complex and made apart over the centuries, extracts a much higher price from the patient to begin with; and/or it has not been appreciated enough that whereas, as a rule, "people are greatly influenced by the environment of which they form part and the role of the environment on the patient's personal life" (Kaufmann et al., 1986), for the hansenian (leprosy patient) not to participate in his environment actively on account of his illness means a profound identity crisis, if not ostracism, even exclusion, from his community; and/or that we have failed to erase once and for all the inhuman image of the disease down to the written word; and/or we have not reached out fully for the patients nor taken into account "their attitudes regarding themselves, their future, and their illness certainly related to the attitudes of those they turn to for help" (Rolston and Chesteen, 1970); and/or we have not been listening enough, or not at all, to the patients, to what they have to say; and/or we have not—and still do—been treating the patients in a way that would have helped them to help themselves, understand and accept their illness, as well as their role as patients; and/or we have not realized that hansenians (leprosy patients)—much moreso than us healthy individuals—yearn for fellowship, restoration of their dignity, their re-insertion in society as has been pointed out.

The Punitive Label

> "More than a fundamental part of how one interacts with people, labels put on people can show one's moral response to them."

The current designation "leprosy" and its cognates or linguistic derivatives—together with their equivalencies in ancient and modern times elaborated by Skinsnes (1974)—is unique in the annals of medicine and world literature, in that it has been—and still is—prone to a host of stereotypes. Never has any other designation given rise to so many pejorative synonyms and/or defamatory connotations.[21]

Never has a designation like this one incurred protest or outcry—past and present—mostly from Western authors.[22] No other designation has been subjected to renewed attempts at change,[23] and known to succeed,[24] with a view to fight stigma attached to it.

Before considering the etymological, social, cultural, ethical, and humane aspects of the issue, a prerequisite is understanding the concept of stigma. Thus, in the first place, one ought to bear in mind that the import of such phenomenon—while inscribed in history—is, as has been observed, determined by a wide range of changing variables within each community of the countries concerned. Or, as Gussow and Tracy (1972) imply, a plausible explanation for stigma is that it "necessarily involves several dimensions on several social and psychological levels." Or put more aptly:

> Stigma is a complex thing. Originally, the word denoted marks made by a pointed instrument or a heated iron. It thus took on the meaning of branding of the skin of man or beast ownership or subjection. It could be a sign of guilt or disgrace, of infamy or shame. More recently, the root etymological meaning has been extended to embrace any departure from a physical norm, or any obvious defect suggestive of a certain condition or disease. A stigma is undesirable, reprehensible, or objectionable. As used in regard to leprosy, stigma refers not only to the characteristic visible signs of paralysis, ulceration, and deformity, associated with advanced peripheral neuropathy, but also by extension of the whole gamut of irrational fears and prejudices under which the leprosy victim suffers.

And again:

> Yet for most people in the Western world, the stigma of leprosy depends less on personal encounters with the condition than on hearsay and folklore. Amongst the educated strata of society, not excepting medical man, a curious dichotomy of thought is frequently observed: there may be a conscious and intellectual acceptance of the scientific facts about leprosy, and at the same time a subconscious rejection of these facts in favor of traditional beliefs. . . . Stigma means cruelty and suffering.

Finally:

> Sir Winston Churchill's fine dictum about crime and criminals might with some justice be adapted to stigma in leprosy: "The mood and

While many other authors have acknowledged since then the erroneous translation of the Old Testament and its nefarious time-honoured impact on Western culture,[27] even though, as intimated by Skinsnes (1964), the attribution of responsibility is widely shared by other cultures elsewhere and not coming under Biblical influence, the likelihood that the "Hebraic reaction to *Tsara'ath* as recorded in the Bible is not so much causative of the social reaction to leprosy as it is a reflection of a response to this unique pathological complex" is to be borne in mind, too.

Nevertheless, *Tsara'ath*, *lepra*, and modern "leprosy" having unrelated meanings, the unfortunate persistent notion in popular imagination that *Tsara'ath* or *lepra* is synonymous with Hansen's disease has a semantic basis only. Those of the influential Biblical tradition admonish Old Testament interpretations of the disease and at the same time accept the Old Testament designation of "leprosy." One could not wish for a more patent contradiction.[28] Besides, preserving still the traditional misrepresentations of "leprosy" on the plea that such a term is embodied anyway in cultures of both endemic and non-endemic countries as suggested by Stringer (1973)—hence implying that nothing can be done about it—is another way to ignore the sensibilities of the hansenian (leprosy patient) and/or his rights as a person.

The case in point as outlined by Rotberg (1975) is that:

> The word "leprosy" has two different connotations. As a synonym for ignominy, defilement, and infamy, it is historically correct and corresponds to the Hebrew Bible's *Tsara'ath*, translated as *lepra* in the Greek Bible. As a medical name, it is illegitimate and derives from the unjustified application of that name to a disease not even known in Moses' time.

Socially

> "Society is judged not by its external achievements, but by the position and meaning it gives to man, by the values it puts on human worth, human dignity, and human conscience."[29]

Society is competitive, writes Skinsnes (1964); furthermore:

When economic conditions in general are poor and the necessities of life are available in only limited quantities, the protection and assistance of the family and group assume an increasing importance to the well-being and survival of the individual. This is demonstrated in China where family connection and influence of friends have traditionally entered into many of life's reactions. When the individual was saddled with the handicap of leprosy and the onus it carries and when in addition, as a result of these concepts, his family and friends abandoned him, the ultimate misfortune had indeed touched him. In the full sense of the saying: "Leprosy has appeared on the face" of both the individual and the social group which so treat him.

Besides, adds the author:

Sharing his community's concepts of leprosy, having heard since childhood the stories current about his disease, and finding no comfort in his religion (for the priest declares his illness a punishment from Heaven and incurable by the gods), the predominant reaction to the person contracting leprosy is one of disgrace and fear. He vehemently protests his innocence of moral delinquency and seeks by all possible means to hide the evidence of his malady.

And again:

One gains the impression that though there is a deep-rooted feeling of revulsion towards leprosy and those suffering from it, the Chinese sense of fate and tolerance enables his society to accept the occurrences of the disease without a preliminary violent reaction. The community approaches the problem of an individual with leprosy with caution. Increasing suspicion is directed at the suspect and gradually his reputation and social position may be completely ruined. This is easily accomplished because society is steeped in accounts and stories having to do with the evidence of persons with leprosy and children are early inculcated with the notion that all such individuals are monsters or creatures of evil.

Finally, the author brings a last touch to the picture when he recalls that:

Added to the concept of religious defilement and of punishment for moral misdemeanor were other accretions and elaborations. Perhaps the most powerful and universal taboos of society are those related to sex, and in the reaction to leprosy as the ultimate in moral delinquency, implications of sexual impropriety were added to the supposed misdemeanor of those afflicted with the loathed and feared condition. Thus Aretaeus speaks of *impulsus ad coitum* and Chinese folklore carries the same implication. The treatment of leprosy is similar to that accorded to adulterers.

Subsequent to Skinsnes's scholarly study of the social aspect of Hansen's disease so greatly influenced by folklore and religion in South China, Antia (1982) brings the point further home when he says that:

In the case of leprosy, where problem of stigma far overrides the problem of technology, our whole approach has been of an almost entirely technical nature. While we have a vast number of medical and paramedical personnel there are hardly any social scientists in the field by which I do not mean social workers. While we spend increasingly more on the scientific aspects of leprosy, including the vaccines, we almost totally ignore research into the equally important social aspects of the disease.

Those with a long experience in the field know only too well lay and professional reactions to disease and patient bordering on the inhuman. In this respect, Haidar (1985) writes that "in most Moslem communities a medieval type of persecution is still practised. The leprosy patient is not accepted as a member of the community and even his family tends to isolate him."[30]

Earlier on, Davey (1968) reports that:

As a patient in society, he is at a particular psychological risk. He inherits community ideas that often associate leprosy with isolation and rejection. These may be astonishingly persistent, even in highly sophisticated societies. Community's attitudes to facial disfigurement make employment present further problems.

Upon the advent of complications inherent in Hansen's disease, Davey concludes that "a vicious circle of psychological trauma is thus initiated, from which few patients are immune."

While Kaufmann et al. (1986) stress once more that the fear of the disease "has remained a part of the characteristic social attitudes toward it right to this day," Rolston and Chesteen (1970), in their broad study of the social, vocational, and psychological problems of Hansen's disease in North America,[31] found out that the patients were most frequently rejected by prospective employers on a pure stigma basis, disturbingly so among health professionals interviewed.

Sankalia (1968) investigated the psychosocial problem under discussion among three thousand unselected hansenians (leprosy patients) in Greater Bombay, and reports that:

> Neither government nor private employers make provision for those who lost their jobs because of leprosy; they are either ignored or segregated by the present legislation.

Gill (1968), in turn, intimates that:

> Since the problems of leprosy patients differ from the problems of the rest of society, their treatment and solution will also differ. History has not been very helpful in the matter. Though their rights as human beings are not different, they are to be given the freedom to exercise them since they are not accepted by society.

Then what asked an anonymous writer?[32] In the light of his experience seemingly in Africa, he has this to say:

> Much depends on the family and on the local feeling. Some patients are from the first excluded from the family, and deprived of possession and inheritance. A few had their children taken away and shared out, like orphans, among relations. The wife might be sent back to her home, possibly in disgrace. In any case, the other members of the family who remained at home shared in the disgrace, and also the fear that they, in turn, might show signs of the disease. In some areas, despite willingness on the part of the healthy members of the family to look after a sick relative, local opinion could be so hostile that he or she was forced to leave, to avoid personal danger and the risk of harm to the rest of the family.

While we cannot but agree with Skinsnes (1964) that social concepts of Hansen's disease are largely influenced, or conditioned, by cultural heritage and mostly those traditional beliefs systems or popular reactions embedded in folklore,[33] subsequently Skinsnes and Elvove (1970) concede that, in both Oriental and Occidental societies, the disease is "set apart as a particular object of horror and opprobrium." The authors acknowledge the long-standing social pathology which has been associated with Hansen's disease, partly through a deficient humanity and lack of rationality. They conclude that:

> For society, the psychological change required is formidable for leprosy, in the historical and literary rather than the medical sense—or better, *Tsara'ath* is deeply embedded in culture and still lies deep in the soul of humanity.

Here again, one subscribes to the above, with the reservation, though, that it should not at this stage prove a deterrent to what can—and should—be done about it in a way to be broached on later.

As already intimated, the hansenian (leprosy patient) feels frequently lonely and isolated on account of his devalued status that makes him so much different from others, a state of affairs because "the patient does not belong any more to the community: he lives as a part of leprosy as a subculture" in the words of Kaufmann et al. (1986). Moreover, the way patients in general are dealt with by the public at large and society in particular would by itself justify considering the disease as first and foremost the person afflicted by it,[34] a view shared by Skinsnes and Elvove (1970), in that the one suffering from Hansen's disease is a personification of that disease. In other words, what popular stance presumably lost in degree, it retained in nature: entrenched secular attitudes compounded of historical, religious, cultural, folkloric, and linguistic implications detrimental still to the patients.

Little doubt, then, that the heavy-loaded past and formidable challenge of the present in relationship to both disease and patient convey another message: unless traditional belief systems or popular stances be forsaken, or the myth and legend about Hansen's disease be broken—as has been advocated—the chances are that the attitudes of the public at large and society in particular will "pursue their arbitrary and dehumanizing whim through time."

In this respect, notwithstanding the intricacies of the above premise, it seems that three additional factors—otherwise seldom, if ever, mentioned—come into play: collective memory of mankind,[35] the ostrich syndrome, and the mentality of our species.

Collective memory, like atavism, is not to be underestimated: it pervades the length and breadth of human affairs that cannot be erased easily. The ostrich syndrome speaks for itself: "most people sense or guess what is at stake or going on, but do not face it squarely. So they pretend that it is neither here nor there." Finally, since "the social reaction to leprosy is a malady rooted in misconceptions and having tendrils extending into antiquity" (Skinsnes, 1964), changing people's minds is in the offing. This may well prove an exercise in futility or an uphill endeavor, unless a more receptive outlook from the public at large and society in particular be gradually brought about, or people's awareness stimulated less with high-toned generalities than sensitized with specifics that would set the issue in its truer perspective, even so with some reservation.

For instance, society in India is stratified into a time-honoured caste system with far-reaching implications as regards attitudes to, and coverage of, the estimated three million plus hansenians (leprosy patients) scattered mostly in the south of that vast subcontinent, and whereby caste, as opposed to class, means that an individual is his proclaimed function solely within it, duties and responsibilities being irrelevant factors in the absence of rewards.[36]

It could never be emphasized enough that research into the comprehensive meaning of the social aspects of Hansen's disease— followed by the widest possible dissemination of its results as has been said—is called for through the co-disciplines of behavioral sciences (social psychology, medical anthropology, sociology, linguistics, and history) as has been suggested,[37] as long as these prove relevant, significant, and applicable to the realities of the disease in both rural and urban areas. This would imply in-depth studies of the social environment in its reactions to the disease (viz. attitudes, practice, beliefs, involvement, provision, communicativeness, semantic problems, etc. as they are linked to that cornerstone of Hansen's disease: stigma).

Culturally

"Ignorance can be harmful. So also complacency, and complacency breeds in a climate of indifference induced by exclusion."

Hansen's disease, the patient, and the current label they share in common have, to a large extent, fallen prey to the whims of myth and legend ingrained in both Occidental and Oriental cultures, in the case of the former partly inspired by erroneous translation of *Tsara'ath* in the Mosaic code and the Greek root word *lepra*, as well as the uncritically accepted Biblical interpretations of the disease in some quarters.

As a result, it is hardly surprising that ancient and modern literature is strewn with liberal use of defamatory overtones pertaining to disease and patient alike, as has already been intimated. In their survey of the use of Hansen's disease in Occidental, non-medical literature, from Dante (1265–1321) to present-day paperbacks, Skinsnes and Elvove (1970) confirm that "this literature uses leprosy as descriptive and representative of almost all imaginable contumely and social opprobrium."

Even though banished from medical literature, the word *leper* is still in vogue in the lay literature of many countries, another example of projection of the traditional belief systems in both scholarly and popular press tantamount to sheer irresponsibility.

The above instances, while proving no doubt counterproductive and counter-educational to this day as reminded by Rotberg (1972, 1973), exert a repeated impact on popular imagination. Besides, contrarily to other communicable diseases, lay dictionaries refer to Hansen's disease in the same vein; so do the arts and media the world over.

The implications are obvious: cultural elements from whatever quarter keep on distorting the image of the disease and, much more seriously, that of the patient as an "embodiment of hopeless physical and moral degradation," hence fuelling popular stance, hence the tendency in some endemic countries to lump hansenians (leprosy patients) into "faceless ghetto minorities."

Unthoughtful attitudes, unwitting reactions, force of habit, irresponsibility altogether inherited from untold generations or not, the ongoing process is verbal, graphic, and visual through representations that are taken literally or symbolically in their intended malignity or not.

What the spoken word does to the public at large and society in particular, the written word achieves for the benefit of the next generation, so far having proved an indictment of the hansenian (leprosy patient) and his disease, thus perpetuating stigma stemming from them both.

Ethically

> "My first concern shall be the welfare of the patient."[38]

No matter how one does look at it—through the inherent equality of rights between one human being to another, or liberalism advocating the universal human—the patient remains in the equation that lends it its legitimacy as such. Patient or not, as Levenstein (1988) has it: "He is first an individual, unique in his thinking, feeling, and behavior. He is dynamic, interacting, and changing with his environment subject to change." For Kaufmann et al. (1986), apart from obvious differences (viz. race, language, culture, and religion), and the diversity of attitudes, feelings, and reactions, each individual patient differs from every other patient, and reacts or responds differently during the various phases of Hansen's disease. Besides, in the view of the authors, doctors, staff members, and auxiliary personnel find themselves in the same situation, and may reject an individual or group by virtue of different social, cultural, and ethical background.

Following the above pertinent observations, Levinsky (1985) emphasizes that physicians are required to attend to the physical and psychological needs of each patient irrespective of other considerations imposed by society. In so doing, one may add, physicians abide by the profession's most noble tradition, while ensuring the rights of health care through a genuine and humane therapeutic approach. The author[39] goes on to say that by deciding how much to do according to what he believes best for the patient, the physician retains his historical single-mindedness role and, in the final analysis, whereas he is the advocate of the patient, the patient in turn remains the true master of the physician. The ideal ethics of the profession would settle for no less.

To what extent the foregoing is relevant to present-day medical practice remains an open question. The issue, here, is quality of health care as much as quality of life demanding certain standards within the contemporary framework reportedly characterized by an ever increasing and costly sophistication of health care, a medical armamentarium growing exponentially, maldistribution of medical manpower, poor adjustment of doctors to actual problems of medicine or, as remarked by Mechanic (1985), "the rapid transformation of medical science and technology in the West, the changing profile and concern of populations, the upsurge of competition among doctors, the fragmentation of medicine and the health professions."

Kriel (1986) has probably the last word when he states that:

> Many problems of contemporary medicine are due to the central biomedical model which, by its very reductionistic nature, offers but an inadequate view of science, disease, and social man.

Besides, what of those "older civilizations where older people keep on cultivating the same old reverence for established ethical norms, in that changes in outlook and behavior from the outside do not penetrate their inner world as if a constant reminder for survival?" What of those equally old religions whereby service is not a concept,[40] when they rather encourage a balancing pragmatism in down-to-earth relationship to, for instance, a most crippling condition like Hansen's disease? What, on the other hand, of the ability to retreat from facts, their implications and consequences; the avoidance of direct evidence; the rejection of concern; the double-think and double-talk as part of a larger scheme in which the ethics of tacit acceptance fits in smugly?

It would, finally, be pertinent to enquire about the attitude of members of the profession not involved in, or concerned by, Hansen's disease: at best marginal, at worst indifferent in the experience of the present writer.

This is particularly reflected in endemic areas where it is felt that should local physicians and health care personnel be, or be made, more aware of the existence of the disease together with its serious implications—while taking the minimum of pains to recognize and diagnose the early signs of Hansen's disease, and referring the patients to the nearest appropriate clinic—control measures of the disease would be greatly enhanced.

Humanely

> *"Homo sum, humani nihil a me alienum puto."*[41]

By the look of it, it would, however tempting, be premature to ask, "Cui bono?"[42] So far, evidence abounds that the fate of the hansenians (leprosy patients) is governed by an interplay of factors (viz. popular stance, societal attitudes, health care, and philanthropy), and forces at work (viz. system, status quo, tradition, conservatism, vested interests, legislation, etc.). The paradox is that, while this interplay of factors and forces at work is no doubt motivated by the best of intentions, the hansenians (leprosy patients) find themselves underprivileged, underclassed, relinquished to a subculture, or alienated on the whole[43]: left with no choice, they are fettered to a most harmful label as well as hostages of stigma, a twin bondage from which release is thought imperative.

Who, then, is to decide for the hansenians (leprosy patients) when their voice is not even heard? Are those advocating the right to speak for them equally committed to the need for redress and retribution in their favor?

Despite the pervading dominance in our cultish time of the subject-to-object or I-it relationship[44] and our Cartesian heritage,[45] the ultimate answer is to be given by the healthy individual of whatever station in life, in that should he subscribe to the virtues of the factors and/or forces at work referred to, then, however remote the chances, however hypothetical the premise, how would he in all honesty—in the event of himself, or kith and kin, contracting the disease—react to the prevailing label "leprosy"?

The Saga of the Name Change

> "The label sticks. The dog is given a bad name,
> whether it deserves it or not. The word 'leper'
> is officially banned: should not 'leprosy' go the
> same way?"[46]

The seeds of the name change were sown a fairly long time ago,
some of them already brought to fruition. They offer no violence to a
state of affairs above established rules, yet remain consistent with
historical, etymological, psychological, social, cultural, ethical, and
humane considerations. The advocacy that the name change be
adopted elsewhere—if not internationally so—could have the
symptoms of a psychoanalytic transfer were it not for what keeps on
sustaining it: its legitimacy. In this respect, a review in chronological
order of how the name change came about warrants attention:

During the Leonard Wood Memorial Conference on Leprosy,
Manila, 1931, the terms *leprosy* and particularly *leper*, having a connotation incompatible with the disease they represent, were the object
of discussions, the general opinion being that a change of name would
be a step to a more reasonable attitude towards the disease on the part
of the public.

The above issue was taken up once more at the Fourth International Leprosy Congress, Cairo, 1938,[47] but to no avail.

It was officially agreed at the Fifth International Leprosy Congress, Havana, 1948, that:

The use of the term "leper" in designation of the patient with leprosy
be abandoned, and the person suffering from the disease be designated
leprosy patient.

The use of any term, in whatever language, which designates a
person suffering from leprosy and to which unpleasant associations are
attached, should be discouraged. However, the use of the name leprosy
should be retained as the scientific designation of the disease. Active
steps should be taken to explain fully to the public its real nature. If the
regional popular use of any less specific terms, in substitution for the
scientific name leprosy, enables the general public to understand more
fully and clearly the advances that have been made in the understanding, diagnosis, and treatment of the disease, such terms may be
used as suitable opportunity offers; but it would be unwise to adopt such

terms to conceal the true nature of the disease. These conclusions should be communicated to scientific journals and the press.

The resolutions regarding the abolition of the term *leper* in favor of the leprosy patients were passed in the course of the Sixth International Leprosy Congress, Madrid, 1953.

The term *hanseniasis* was officialized by the Secretariat for Health, São Paulo state, Brazil, in 1967, in respect to all documents and correspondence of the Public Health Service.

The following year, the Assembly of deputies of that state approved the new designation *Departmento de Dermatologia Sanitaria* instead of *Departmento de Profilaxia da Lepra.*

Programs under the aegis of the WHO/Pan-American Health Organization, Guadalajara, Mexico, recommended that studies and tests be undertaken to overcome the lack of prompt and effective results obtained until then with the procedures in use in health education and public information on the leprosy problem. A group of participants held that one of their difficulties had to do with the term "leprosy," and recommended the possibility of modification, a move approved by the subsequent Seventeenth Brazilian Congress of Hygiene, Salvador.

The Seminar of Leprosy (Hanseniasis) Control, held in the course of the Eighteenth Brazilian Congress of Hygiene, São Paulo, 1970, reached the conclusion that a new terminology would facilitate health education and control of the disease and contribute to eliminate the social stigma hanging over the patients and their families.

The Technical Administrative Council, Public Health Service, São Paulo, considered improper the utilization of the term *lepra* to designate the infection caused by *M. leprae* from both a social and control standpoint, hence the designation hanseniasis from then on. Responding to an appeal of 117 signatories from fifteen countries, the Council of the International Leprosy Association (ILA), following the Tenth International Leprosy Congress, Bergen, 1973, acknowledged the problems caused by the term "leprosy" and consequently advised that countries were free to adopt other terminology of their choice.

The then president of the Italian Republic approved in 1974 the new law promulgated by both Chamber of deputies and Senate forbidding the use of the terms *lebbra, lebbrosario*, and any other derivatives of *lebbra*, such terms to be replaced by *Morbo di Hansen, hanseniano, colonia, or instituto hanseniano*, or any derivative of the name Hansen.

The former president of Brazil officially decreed in 1975 that the National Division of Leprosy and the National Campaign against Leprosy be henceforth designated Division of Public Health Dermatology and National Campaign against Hanseniasis respectively. In the same year, the new rules and regulations of the U.S. Public Health Service were drastically revised, and as a result Hansen's disease was substituted for "leprosy," an official move at least in the regulations, pending approval from the U.S. Senate.

During the National Conference for the Appraisal of the Control Policy for Hanseniasis, Brasilia, in 1976, the Cultural Barriers Group reached the conclusion that the introduction of the new terminology at the national level was a first step for a change of the stigmatization concept of the disease, and for the eventual removal of cultural barriers.

The term *lepra* and its derivatives were proscribed by decree of the Ministry of Health, Brazil. In the same year, the foundation of the College of Hansenology of Endemic Countries, Brazil, took place, and the *Associação Brasileira de Leprologia* had its designation changed to *Associação Brasileira de Hansenologia*.

By decree of the Ministry of Social Affairs, Portugal, the term Hansen's disease was officially proposed in 1977 to replace the current one. The designation "Institute of Assistance to Lepers" was replaced by the Assistance of Hansen's Disease Patients.

The Workshop on Human Aspects in the Treatment of Leprosy Patients, Eleventh International Leprosy Congress, Mexico City, 1978, stipulated that the word leprosy be used "with caution since it tends to have a socio-historical, in addition to a medical connotation." In the same year, the *Departamento de Lucha contra la Lepra* was renamed *Departamento de Sanitaria Dermatologica* with a view to banish the pejorative term *lepra*.

The 1978 Edition in Portuguese of the International Classification of Diseases, WHO, adopted the term Hanseniasis besides *Doenca de Hansen* and *Infecção por Mycobacterium leprae*, the term *lepra* not appearing any more among the synonyms.

The Synod of the Presbyterian Church in the Cameroon, West Africa, had the name "Leprosy Hospital" changed to Hanseniasis and Rehabilitation Centre. The National Division of Epidemiology of the

Bolivian Ministry of Social Welfare and Public Health adopted in 1979 the new terminology in its Manual of Technical Norms and Administrative Procedures for the Control of Hansen's Disease.

The Trinidad and Tobago Hansen's Disease Control Unit was mentioned as such in its annual report of that year. In Jamaica, the designation Hansen's disease was officially adopted by the Ministry of Health. In 1981, the Leprosy Control Programme in Guyana was changed to Hansen's Disease Control Programme. Publication by the WHO/Pan-American Health Organization in 1983 of a booklet in Portuguese entitled *Manual para o Control de Hanseniase*.

Hanseniasis is mentioned as one of the synonyms for leprosy in the International Nomenclature of Diseases (1st Ed., Vol. 11, CIOMS and WHO, Geneva, 1985).

Judging from the foregoing, the official name change carries more weight in endemic than in non-endemic countries as expected, with the intended purpose to destigmatize an overloaded situation in which the hansenians (leprosy patients) are caught, yet it would be futile—to the point of overrating human nature—to bank on quick returns or positive feedback.

Official implementation of the name change in question is one thing in theory, quite another one in practice when it comes to achieving concrete results since it spells long-term policy backed up by far-reaching media coverage over, more likely than not, decades.

A case in point of late is Brazil, in that it is not surprising to hear from Oliveira et al. (1989) that, following the first six months of a multimedia campaign "both society and government circles were inclined to underplay the problem." The idea, in this case, is to pursue that line of action, as long as the medium is indeed proving the message.

The Workable Alternative

> The worthiness of a cause enhanced by the facts relies in the short term on neither gain nor loss. Its recognition and universal acceptance lie in the long run instead.

Little wonder that the historical, etymological, psychological, social, cultural, ethical, and humane facets of the designation *leprosy* and its cognates, carried by their logical momentum one way or another, lead to the name change in some countries so far.

Yet, even though bent on remedial purposes by virtue of its calling, the name change is proving at odds with most Western and non-Western tradition and present mentality. Be it as it may: the issue is central to the concept of a much overdue retribution and redress[48] in favor of the hansenians (leprosy patients). As the main correlate of that issue, a campaign of destigmatization extended to medical, paramedical, social, religious, and educational institutions is advocated by Dogliotti (1979).

Prior to the implementation of the name change in the countries and institutions referred to, literature pertaining to the issue is well documented, the "whole shades of grey of the controversy" testifying, if nothing else, to the "tremendous impact of the current terminology and uniqueness of the disease" as pointed out by Rotberg (1974).

Enquiring from the start—as is being done still—(i) what good a name change would accomplish, (ii) what advantage(s) would it bring, or (iii) whether it would directly result or play a significant role in removing the stigma attached to the disease as has been altogether expressed, would prove premature. Rather, the critical appraisal of the main objections to the name change is called for. Thus:

> Why bring up an ancient movement against the appellation leprosy, an issue which has been discussed over and over again . . . when the International Leprosy Association has turned down this name change in the past and despite some twenty years of agitation on a worldwide basis, most physicians engaged in leprosy work are not in favor of the change for a number of reasons (Skinsnes, 1971).

The aforesaid movement has since then proved fruitful in some countries. The die is cast in favor of those hansenians (leprosy patients) living there, and hope remains for the others elsewhere, (i) not so much to rectify an affront to one's sense of rightness or fair play nor (ii) inveighing against abuses of the past and continued errors of the present, but (iii) because one has, perhaps, become entrapped in ready-made formulas at the expense of the obvious or (iv) that, at the limit, one needs a psychological crutch to be tided over the evidence of it all.

> The term leprosy, and its recognizable variants, is limited to those few languages which are primarily prevalent in areas of low, or virtually no leprosy incidence. . . . For most of the Orient and Africa where leprosy is a distinct public health problem, this specific name change is meaningless and even unintelligible to that segment of the population where folklore is most deeply rooted (Skinsnes, 1964).

However correct these observations, it is equally a question of perspective anew, in keeping with the Zeitgeist or spirit of the present time, in that once the principle of the name change is accepted in good faith—and not to suit "academic purism" instead—the local equivalencies of the word "leprosy"—however embedded they may be the world over—could be dealt with in the vernacular by means of appropriate health education modalities and multi-media campaigns.

> As long as leprosy remains the world's greatest crippling and deforming disease, its fear and horror will continue irrespective of its designation (Skinsnes, 1971).

It is one thing to be crippled by, say polio or rheumatoid arthritis, and quite another to be the deformed victim of Hansen's bacillus (*M. leprae*) since the latter bears the unmistakable stamp of what the members of the community are never fooled by. As Warren (1972) observes: "Persons with marked disabilities of many types from causes other than leprosy appear to be fully accepted by their fellow men." In other words, never in the case of Hansen's disease.

> The name change is neither valid nor pertinent to the rest of the world, and would not affect millions of patients whose languages are not English and have their own deep embedded terminology and folklore related to this disease, this folklore totally unrelated to the Biblical use of leprosy (Skinsnes, 1971).

With the permutation of values in our rapidly changing world, the tantalizing conundrum why and/or how convince people to the contrary need not apply anymore. The rationale behind the workable alternative submitted in this section can be translated in the vernacular, with a view to (i) democratize Hansen's disease and (ii) release the patients from the bondage of stigma.

The aversion for the use of eponyms in scientific circles.

This is quite understandable and, in fact, legitimate. Yet, in light of the present issue, what does the alleged inconvenience of an eponym weigh, furthermore, in fault of a better term? When even an eponym is preferable to a name that makes patients with modern "leprosy" go into hiding, and unable to save their families from ostracism as well or secure employment even after cure as Lendrum (1952) and so many authors have pointed out since then?

The new terminology would be too confusing to the medical world, the existence of two or more terminologies difficult for doctors to communicate (Skinsnes, 1971).

Not necessarily so on the strength of the alternate terminology used in the present monograph, when more so applicable stepwise.

There would never be a 100% acceptance (Jopling, 1983).

Quite likely so, yet neither a deterrent nor an impediment per se. In that sort of endeavor made explicit so far, one does not try to gather the *consensus omnium* in the first place, but go ahead while building and/or maintaining the evidence for it, should it be for the benefit of the next generation of hansenians (leprosy patients) instead.

Clinically, the new terminology an unsolvable dilemma.

An ambiguous, if not misleading, statement since dilemma means "a situation necessitating a choice between two equally undesirable alternatives, or a problem that seems incapable of a solution." On the other hand, if the author implies *on the horns of dilemma*, it would spell "facing the choice between two equal alternatives or an awkward situation." This semantic digression is intended since, as shown below, the alternate terminology used in the present monograph entails neither an unsolvable problem nor an awkward situation for that matter, but affords its own logicality based on the complete removal of the root word *lepra* and its cognates so as to be consistent throughout. Hence:

Current Terminology	Suggested Terminology
Leprosy	Hansen's disease
Leprology	Hansenology
Leprologist	Hansenologist
Leprosy patient	Hansenian
Mycobacterium leprae	Hansen's bacillus or, better still, *Mycobacterium hansenii*
Tuberculoid leprosy (TT)	Polar Paucibacillary form (PP)
Tuberculoid patient	Paucibacillary patient
Borderline tuberculoid (BT)	Borderline paucibacillary (BP)
Borderline tuberculoid patient	Borderline paucibacillary patient
Epithelioid cell granuloma or tubercle	Immunological granuloma
Lepromatous leprosy (LL)	Polar multibacillary form (PM)
Lepromatous patient	Multibacillary patient
Borderline lepromatous (BL)	Borderline multibacillary (BM)
Borderline lepromatous patient	Borderline multibacillary patient
Lepromatous infiltration	Macrophage infiltration
Leproma	Non-immunological or macrophage granuloma
Lepra cells	Virchow's cells
Erythema nodosum leprosum (ENL)	Erythema nodosum hansenicum (ENH)
Lepromin	Mitsuda's Antigen
Leprostatic	Hansenostatic
Leprous, leprotic	Hansenic
Leproid	Hansenoid
Leprid (e)	Hansenid (e)
Leprosarium	Hansen's disease hospital

"The name change will neither fool society nor change its attitudes" (Skinsnes, 1971). Earlier on, the author observes that "Unfortunately society will want to know what Hansen's disease (or Hanseniasis) is. Recognizing it as leprosy, will then need the same rational explanation for its misconceptions that it should be challenged immediately with the same energetic efforts that are applied to promoting the attempted name change" (1964).

Convit (1973) enjoins that "The evasive term 'hanseniasis' to most minds calls for an explanation and when it is identified with traditional leprosy it is apt to impress the mind more poignantly than would be the case when the disease is called by its current name."

Both of the above remarks fit into what has been dubbed the "duck test": "No matter what leprosy is called, if it looks like leprosy and sounds like leprosy, people will perceive it as leprosy!" The argument is no longer tenable in the light of historical, psychological, etymological, social, cultural, ethical, and humane considerations expounded in favor of the name change, let alone the fact that, in the meantime, some countries and institutions have adopted that change without indulging in explanations for the sake of the public at large and society in particular. While it is gratifying to hear from Skinsnes (1971) that: "It must, of course, be recognized that the emotionalism of the appeal (for the name change) is based on a justifiable, and commendable, deep anger at the injustices and irrationality of society's opprobrium," it is neither emotionalism nor anger to that extent. Rather, the timely evidence that the aforesaid society is, in fact, the villain in that it has been extracting for too long too high a price from the patient, the disease, and the label that they share in common.

> The doctor is in a difficult situation when the patient asks: "You tell me that I am suffering from hanseniasis. What is it?"
> If in answering this question, the doctor answers "leprosy," then nothing has been gained.
> If, on the other hand, in answering this question, the doctor avoids the word "leprosy," the patient is unlikely to persist with treatment once he sees clinical improvement. (Jopling, 1983).

When, as in the above case, the patient is unaware that he has contracted the disease and ought, therefore, to be told about it, the aim of the exercise would be to depolarize or defuse a situation before the patient is entrapped in it, i.e. to the point of personalizing a disease that much set apart as a result of social pathology. Remedial measures could be applied to such a situation upon the understanding that the medium proves the message. Hence the above patient could be told instead: "You have Hansen's disease, named after the Norwegian doctor who discovered the cause for it, and while your chances of getting completely cured are excellent in the short run, your treatment must be quite regular since the penalty for neglect is high. Your disease has for centuries been very wrongly identified with the 'leprosy' (or *lèpre, Aussatz, Spedalked, Lova, Kusth, Ma-feng, Akushitu,* etc.) spoken of by society and the media, a term at any rate on its way out."

The foregoing evokes, admittedly, an ideal situation when the patient is educated and cooperative and society more tolerant. It would, arguably, prove the exception to the rule. Yet, either way, it would mean a major step ahead if followed by the members of the profession, paramedical and health care personnel for a start, with supportive health education and multi-media approach in the community where the patient lives since, otherwise, it could prove self-defeating. As regards patients already affected by Hansen's disease—moreso in the advent of disability and/or deformity—a similar message in the vernacular, backed up with health education and media referred to, would equally apply upon the injunction that hansenians (leprosy patients) learn about their disease and fight stigma on its own ground.

Finally,

"There is a case for retaining the substance of current terminology related to leprosy, particularly because of fund raising" (Stringer, 1973).

Fund raising in favor of Hansen's disease and those afflicted by it embodies a paradoxical situation, in that its main source of revenue is from the public at large and society in particular who, incidentally, having alienated disease and patient alike throughout history, seemingly assuage their guilt complex by providing significantly to the treatment and welfare of, admittedly, thousands of patients, and share appreciably in the research program of the disease as has been submitted. On the other hand, it has been stressed that removal of the term "leprosy" would seriously jeopardize the dynamics of fund raising and, by the same token, threaten the very existence of many philanthropic organizations themselves. What is more, to the sponsors and administrators of these organizations, once the principle has been secured for so long by the system and uncritically accepted by the medical profession itself, well, it just cannot be corrected.

Arguably, a situation can be corrected if the repeal for specific measures be converted into the opposite principle with modifications if need be. In the case of Hansen's disease, it spells a justified need, let alone a precedent created in other parts of the world. It embodies good faith, if not fair play, when it comes to restore human sensitivities overlooked and/or ignored for so long by the public at large and society in particular. With equal cogency, secularization of Hansen's disease—shorn of divine displeasure or punishment and morality as has been advocated—is a contemporary reality, at least in the West. It follows that philanthropic organizations could relate their publicity to the demands of the situation if the text of their appeal for funds—while retaining its credibility and substance—be amended accordingly.

It would seem that the overall issue pertaining to this section has been prone to more difference in conceptual levels and entrenched views than divergence of opinion and room for openness of mind. Moreover, the overall implications are clear: (i) the classical or traditional representation of "leprosy" and "leprosy patient" is only credible as long as people propagating it believe in their propagation without the benefit of critical scrutiny; and (ii) the evidence so far that no amount of education, persuasion, or enticement will suffice to throw off the shackles of the past as long as the current designations "leprosy" and "leprosy patient" are not replaced by another designation free of the possibility of stigmatization.

The accumulation of historical, psychological, etymological, social, cultural, ethical, and humane evidence pointing to the rationale behind the advocacy of the name change does, at the same time, "recall nothing even remotely like it, nothing that would bear comparison as parallel or precedent in the annals of human endeavor."

It means that the magnitude of the issue cannot be confined any longer to the whims of sheer rationality nor be "frozen" by mere institutional decree or the revindications of ossified policy: the onus, it would seem, rests on Western medicine, those of the influential Biblical persuasion, and authorities directly involved with Hansen's disease, notwithstanding those non-Western countries where similar attitudes prevail and current equivalencies of the word "leprosy" are loaded terms.

What is at stake is a commitment to, involvement with, and concern for the hansenians (leprosy patients) matched by their inherent right to integrity, dignity, and humaneness, i.e., a subject-to-subject relationship in the Buberian sense, yet devoid of highbrow compassion and discriminatory connotation appertaining to his condition.

The purpose of the exercise is, as Lendrum (1952) puts it, that: "The avoidance of tragic misunderstandings is far more important than adherence to artificial standards of linguistic purism." And in the words of Dogliotti (1979):

> A creative approach in the process of education and training in the disease has become essential if we really wish hanseniasis to emerge as a disease like any other. All efforts intended to control the disease are inescapably destined to fail unless the significance of stigma and allied socio-economic factors realize that we are dealing with human beings. In order to fight against terror, taboos and misinformation, we must move away from the opprobrious term "leprosy" and replace it with the eponym hanseniasis.

The goal is to (i) liberate the hansenians (leprosy patients) from the stereotypes of their condition, the "endless self-defeating immobilities" nurtured by the public at large and society in particular; and (ii) open the way so that the disease will stand on its own, once its designation and linguistic variants will have been done away with.

One cannot help thinking that, had the name of Hansen as the discoverer of the etiological agent been equally honoured as those of Pasteur, Lister, Donovan, Leishman, Bruce, Candid, Ricketts, etc.,[49] things would have in all likelihood been different, if not made easier nowadays. In effect, Feldman (1953), while admitting not being a microbiologist nor posing for an authority either, is in favor of having a less opprobrious term than "leprosy" providing it had a taxonomic basis. Thus:

> As well known, the microorganism generally accepted as the causative agent of leprosy is an acid-alcohol-fast organism discovered by Hansen, a Norwegian physician, in 1868. The biological characteristics of this organism require its classification under the family Mycobacteriaceae, where it is correctly placed under the genus Mycobacterium. . . . The objectionable feature, and the obstacle that must be surmounted in

considering a change in nomenclature, is the name of the species, which is leprae. As a way around this difficulty, the name of the species might be changed from leprae to hansenii (in the name of Hansen who discovered the organism). The name of the organism, then, might become officially Mycobacterium hansenii.

It would have been quite fitting to submit Feldman's proposal to the Judicial Commission of the International Committee on Bacterial Nomenclature for approval. Yet to the best knowledge of the present writer, no concerted move to that effect has been officially made, notwithstanding redressing a blatant injustice in memory of Hansen. Such redress, however belatedly, would no doubt help in paving the way to the advocated name change elsewhere in the world.

One is aware that, in practice, the advocated name change elsewhere in the world would most probably be going against the grain of tradition belief systems or conservatism, hence the anticipation or likelihood that (i) The evidence for it might be unwillingly acknowledged, or treated as something outside the field of one's experience. (ii) The whole matter might not be given due importance, hence not worthy of new recognition. (iii) Not facing the issue would be easier, less troublesome, or more sensible to maintain the status quo. (iv) The final solution might be paved with assumed or imagined obstacles, efforts coming to naught anyway. (v) Or a weak collective response might be the case, persistent enough as unavowed excuse for inaction as altogether pointed out.

In the final analysis, after all that has been elaborated and commented so far, it would seem that, irrespective of the foregoing, the ins and outs of the advocated name change will require a quantum leap out of the ordinary, a mobilization of good will and mass cooperation, if called upon to be implemented elsewhere in the world.

While it is easy to draw a plan of action of this magnitude, however thoughtful or authoritative, it is feared that such a plan is doomed to failure unless "forged with the fellowship of understanding" at all levels concerned, and met with foresight and forbearance, if not fortitude.

In short, such a plan of action would mean a transitional umbrella program[50] that will unavoidably meet with debits and hurdles, yet at the same time "symbolize a way to the future leaving out the greatest options in the service" of the hansenians (leprosy patients) them-selves.[51]

Notes

1. Remark of the present writer (1967).
2. McDougall and Yamalkar (1987) went as far as saying that "The treatment of leprosy sufferers throughout history is one of the darkest examples of man's inhumanity to man."
3. A disease quite familiar to the present writer, in light of his experience in, namely, Gambia (West Africa), Nigeria, Upper Burma, India (Andhra Pradesh), Zaïre Republic, Southern Sudan, and Natal (RSA).
4. WHO Advisory Committee on Health Research: Health Research Strategy, Geneva, 1986.
5. Malaria holds the world record: a reported 200 million new victims every year, and thousands of deaths.
6. According to the WHO, gastroenteritis is responsible for one third of the deaths of children aged five and less; an estimated five million of these children die annually.
7. Browne (1979, 1985 and 1985); Skinsnes (1964 and 1970).
8. Languillon (1986) adds that "The Hebrews were not the originators of such a concept, its causal sin being already found in Leviticus, the oral tradition of India, as well as the Egyptian and Chinese manuscripts" (cf. the present writer's translation).
9. Tas (1983).
10. Davey (1968) reminds us that "In our scientific concern with leprosy, we must not forget the patient as a person, and the profound influence upon him of the imponderable psychological factors that are specially associated with his disease." Earlier on, Ryrie (1951)—probably the first among Western authors to delve into the subject—singled out a common denominator among three groups of patients and people connected with the disease, namely irrational fear tied up with a sense of shame and disgust or sprung from a sort of guilt complex in the form of punishment. Besides, taking an extreme view, Ryrie doubted whether mankind had evolved enough to take care of the victims of chronic diseases! In his study of the genesis of "Lepra-Angst" among Chinese patients, Skinsnes (1969) finds a simliar common denominator and remarks that "Lepra-Angst" is identified as "the guilt-fear of individuals who, not having leprosy, believe themselves to be so afflicted."
11. Flynn and Harvey (1968).
12. Munoz and Storkan (1968).
13. Campos et al. (1978).
14. D'Almeida et al. (1986).
15. Viz. his life work, interests, needs, problems, etc.
16. Let alone that he lives in a world where, by and large, preventive medicines, health care, and social welfare, not being a productive sector of the economy, do not figure on the priority list. On the other hand, scarcity of resources, shortcom-

ings of nutrition and sanitation, poverty, etc., do provide a vicious circle whereby the least privileged of the community pay a higher price for it.

17. I.e., as opposed to humiliation (Albert Camus, 1913–1960). In this respect, the hansenian (leprosy patient) could always shoot back to us: "You have not paid with the price of your own dignity. How, then, can you truly communicate with those who like us did?" (George Steiner in *George Steiner: A Reader* [1986].)

18. Or, as Lechat (1981) remarks, the hansenian (leprosy patient) "is an expiatory victim, the healthy members of the community exorcising their fear of death by using the disease for propitiatory purposes, hence making the patient guilty of his own illness."

19. By the same token—and to paraphrase George Steiner—are we not thus emptying of their humanity those hansenians (leprosy patient) whom we shun, deny care, and deprive of the right to be heard? By doing so, are we not making them redundant, even naked?

20. Dr. Margaret Brand cited by Pfytche (1981).

21. Viz. "vice," "sin," "filth," "loathsomeness," "corruption," "dirtiness," "ignominy," "repulsiveness," "disgust," "defilement," "infamy," etc.

22. As mostly quoted by Rotberg (1972 and 1973):

   "A common cause for suicide and crime" (Souza, 1940). "A curtain of terror"; "a disastrous barrier to good medical care and public health measures"; "a historical misnomer" (Lendrum, 1945 and 1952). "An ugly name" (Faget, 1947). "A shame for the patient and his family" (Lichtwardt, 1948). "Ignominious" (Feldmann, 1953). "A disintegrator of the patient's personality" (Letayf, 1955). "The most stigmatizing and antisocial word" (Rabello, 1955).

   "A horror based on a confusion of ideas" (Gramberg, 1960). "A name that has to be changed urgently" (Swellengrebel, 1960). "A nightmare, a terrible shock" (Diniz, 1965). "The malignancy that seems to accompany it" (Quiroga, 1968). "The most negative of all medical terms" (Rolston and Chesteen, 1970). "Associated with medieval darkness and millenary malediction and superstition" (Becker, 1971).

   "A label that blocks education" (Mangiaterra, 1972). "It annihilates all attempts at public enlightenment, as it is loaded with ancient emotional charge of rejection, constantly reinforced by all communication media"; "a label of primary force"; "counter-educational and counterproductive" (Rotberg, 1972, 1973, 1974, and 1982). "A continued psychic pain and trauma" (1974). "A traditional stigmatizing and detrimental connotation" (Dogliotti, 1979).

23. Viz. Hansen's disease (Lichtwardt, 1948); Hansenosis (Feldman, 1953) and Goldman (1963); Mycobacterial Neurodermatosis (Ross Innes, 1963); Morbus Hansen (Rabello, 1970); Hanseniasis (Baruffa and Dogliotti, 1979).

24. Cf. Brazil Hansen's Disease Centre, Carville (U.S. Public Health Service), Portugal (Ministry of Social Welfare), Costa Rica, Bolivia (Ministry of Social Affairs and Public Health), Jamaica, Guyana, Italy, Trinidad and Tobago, Cape Vert.

25. Editorial, *Leprosy Review* 43 (1972): 69–72.

26. First adequately described by Danielson and Boeck in 1847 as intimated, specifically defined by Hansen in 1874, and only since then has had its present official meaning as remarked by Lendrum. In fact, as Browne (1985) puts it: "Nothing of note seems to have added to the medieval corpus of knowledge of diverse clinical manifestations of low-resistant leprosy until the publication of *Om Spedalsked.*"

27. As admitted by Lowe (1942), MacArthur (1953), Cochrane (1956), Gramberg (1959), Nida (1960), and Wellington (1961), quoted by Skinsnes (1964).
28. Cf. the remarks of Cochrane (1970): "Through a mistranslation of *Zara'ath*, the word leprosy has a most unfortunate sinister connotation." Skinsnes (1970) enjoins upon saying that "The problem of leprosy and *tsara'ath* has not been essentially improved and that obfuscation has been increased in connection with the new translation of the English Bible."
29. To speak of society in general implies a notion akin to abstraction, yet society in particular—as is presently the case vis-à-vis Hansen's disease—has, by contrast, its own different and deep-rooted belief systems providing it with whatever is significant and/or relevant to it as has been pointed out. Apart from the "inadequate opportunity structure attributed to society," one is reminded by Prof. Jeffrey Grey, London Institute of Psychiatry, that "Society is not a human invention, it is mammalian, yet a whole breed of scientists who ought to know better speak as if 'society' is human and 'biology' pre-human."

    From a more explicit viewpoint as expounded by Belgian philosopher Grynpas (1967): "Society is not just a group of individuals in search of their destiny. It is equally a place or locus of daily life made up essentially of human relationship . . . not in reciprocity to exist, but to be, i.e., to be justified. Such human relationship bears on the immediate recognition of other people, in that they are my fellow-men, a reflection of myself. A necessary relationship, indeed, because it conveys to my conscience and immediate sense of common touch, a sense of my own importance, as a result of which communication assumes a dimension whereby my fellow-men and myself meet one another." (In *La Philosophie*, Marabout Université, 1967; translation by the present writer.)
30. Isolation here spells "leprosy" villages or "leprosaria"-like camps still in existence. The present writer has known numerous instances whereby individual hansenians (leprosy patients) were forced to live in a separate hut well outside their villages, and left on their own.
31. Namely California, Texas, New York City, Florida, Louisiana, and Puerto Rico, involving 252 patients intensely interviewed.
32. A Medical Man, "The Stigma of Leprosy—A Personal Experience," *Leprosy Review* 43 (1972): 83–84.
33. I.e., the written literature of a people expressed in its traditional beliefs, customs, idioms, tales, music, etc.
34. "La lèpre, c'est l'homme!" (Dr. Frans Hemerijckx).
35. Or that "medium from nostalgia and hope to conservatism and blindness."
36. Cf. V.S. Naipaul, who went further in saying that "Caste, sanctioned by the Gita with an almost propagandistic fervor, might be seen as part of older Indian pragmatism, the 'life' of classical India. It has decayed and ossified with society, and its corollary, function, has become all. . . . Every man is an island; each man to his function, his private contract with God. This is the realization of the Gita's selfless action. This is caste. In the beginning a no doubt useful division of labour from social obligation, position from duties. It is inefficient and destructive; it has created a psychology which will frustrate all improving plans" (in *An Area of Darkness*, 8th Ed., 1984).
37. Pre-Congress Workshop, *Leprosy Review* 59 (1968): 284–307.
38. Part of the Hippocratic Oath.
39. Quoting Fried (1975) and Hiatt (1975) as well.
40. "And do thy duty, even it be humble, rather than another's even if it be great. To

die in one's duty is life; to live in another's is death," as it applies still to the Gita's preaching degree of one's station in life whilst at the same time a call to self-fulfillment in the words of V.S. Naipaul (1984).

41. "I am a man, nothing touching man is alien to me." (cf Terence, Latin poet and comedy-writer, Carthage, second century A.D.).

42. To whom does it benefit?

43. Tied up with the remarks of Dogliotti (1979), i.e., "Latent segregation, obsolete legislation, deficient health education, sensationalism, misguided charity," though up to a point.

44. Expressed by Martin Buber (1878–1965), renowned Vienna-born philosopher of the Hasidic tradition. Or, in view of the present writer, the perpetuation of man-as-object, or mere statistical unit way down the human hierarchy.

45. From which stems the dichotomy of mind and body at the biological, psychological, and cultural levels: man as dichotomized individual or depersonalized social being as has been submitted.

46. Editorial, *Leprosy Review* 43 (1972): 69–72.

47. The first International Leprosy Congress was held in 1897, Berlin; the second one in 1909, Bergen; the third one in Strassbourg, 1923.

48. Retribution and redress are not just products of human consciousness, in that, as has been observed, both spring from their own foundation that had been laid down beforehand. Or, perhaps, as proposed by the present writer, from a sense of justice. But then "Human justice is seldom at home," or, to quote Lord Balfour, "There is not enough of it to go around."

49. Viz. pasteurellosis, listerellosis, leishmaniasis, donovanosis, brucellosis, candidiasis, rickettsiosis, etc.

50. While there is little doubt that the hardest nuts to crack spell traditional belief systems in the guise of conservatism, skepticism, professionalism, and bureaucratic resistance, it would seem that the keys to that program in both endemic and partially endemic areas are: (i) Reaching out for all people at community level. (ii) Presenting in the vernacular facts relating to the hansenian (leprosy patient) in perspective anew (viz. historical, psychological, etymological, social, ethical, and humane considerations as simplified and briefly as possible). (iii) Arousing and sustaining community motivation with concurrent multi-communication media. (iv) Identifying obstacles and clarifying the way(s) they could be bypassed or removed. (v) Ensuring the continuity of the program within a climate conducive to community awareness, and gradual change of outlook towards the patient and his disease.

51. In keeping with what the present writer expressed in 1971: "We as medical men, owe humanely, morally, and professionally such a breakthrough (viz. the name change) to the millions of hansenians who, in other parts of the world—to use the words of a well-known hansenologist—are the victims of an acid-fat bacillus made more virulent by ignorance, prejudice and fear."

References

Antia, H.H. Leprosy: Primary Health Care: The Mandwa Project. *Lep. Rev.* 53 (1982): 205–209.

Baruffa, G. Let's Call it Hanseniasis. *Hans. Int'l* (1979), 2:115.

Bloom, B.R. Towards a Leprosy Vaccine. *World Health*, May, 1985, 3–5.

Brand, P.W. Neuropathic Ulceration: Deformities of the Hands and Feet in Leprosy. Europ. Lep. Symp., Genoa, 1981. Hlth. Coop. Pprs. 1 (1982): 93–127.

Browne, S.G. Leprosy in Europe: Epidemiology and Residual Foci. *Lep. Rev.* 50 (1979): 84–86.

———. Social and Vocational Rehabilitation of Leprosy Patients in Asia. ILO/DANIDA Asian Regional Seminar, Bombay, 1981.

———. LEPROSY, Documenta Geigy, Acta Clinica, 1984.

———. The History of Leprosy. In *Leprosy*, ed. R.C. Hastings, Churchill Livingstone, 1985, 1–14.

Brubaker, M.L. Leprosy: Fifty Years of Progress. Rpr. Bol. Offic. Sanit. Panamericana (English Ed.) 6 (1972): 1–14.

Bryceson, A.D.M. Immunology. Europ. Lep. Symp., Genoa, 1981/ Hlth Coop. Pprs 1 (1982): 33–38.

Campos, F.J. et al. The Mental Status of the Leprosy Patient. *Proc. XI Int'l Lep. Cong. Mexico City*, 1978, Excerpta Medica Amsterdam-Oxford-Princeton. *J. Lep.* 38 (19760): 207–209.

Convit, J. Editorial, *Int. J. Lep.* 43 (1973): 112–117.

Dogliotti, M. Leprostigma in Hanseniasis *South African Med. J.* 55 (1979): 102–103.

D'Almedia et al. Le Hansènien Face à son angoisse. *Acta Lep.* IV (1986), I: 59–72.

Del Cerro, S.G. The Patient-Doctor Relationship in Leprosy. *Int. J. Lep.* 36 (1968); Abstr. Cong. Pprs. XIII 156: 634.

Davey, T.F. The Leprosy Patient and His Illness. *Int. J. Lep.* 36 (1968); Abstr. Cong. Pprs. XIII 153: 633.

Ell, S.R. Plague and Leprosy in the Middle Ages: A Paradoxical Cross-Immunity? Editorial, *Int. J. Lep.* 55 (1987): 345.

Feldman, W.H. Hansenosis for Leprosy. Correspondence, *JAMA* 152 (1953), 11: 100.

Fytche, T.J. The Eye in Leprosy. Editorial, *Lep. Rev.* 52 (1981): 111–119.

Fleming, S. The Leper's Dilemma. Current Lit. *Int. J. Lep.* 57 (1989): 127.

Flynn, P.E. and Harvey H. Investigation of the Psychological World of the Hansen's Disease Patient. *Int. J. Lep.* 36 (1968); Abstr. Cong. Pprs. XIII 155: 633.

Gill, I.K. Social Problems of Leprosy Patients. *Int'l J. Lep.* 36 (1968); Abstrc. Cong. Papers XIII 158: 635.

Goldman, L. Letter to the Editor. *Lep. Rev.* 35 (1963): 51–52.

Gussow, Z. and Tracy, S. Stigma and the Leprosy Phenomenon—a Socio-Medical Perspective. *Int. J. Lep.* 36 (1968); Abstr. Cong. Pprs. XIII 151: 632.

———. The Phenomenon of Leprosy Stigma in Continental United States. *Lep. Rev.* 43 (1972): 85–93.

Haidar, A.A.M. Leprosy: the Moslem Attitude. *Lep. Rev.* 56 (1985): 17–21.

Hastings, R.C. The 1987 Journal—A Continuing Perspective. *Int. J. Lep.* 56 (1988): 82–100.

Jopling, W.H. On the Question of Terminology: Letter to Prof. A. Rotberg published in the *Star*, Nov.–Dec., 1983.

Kaufmann, A. et al. The Social Dimension of Leprosy. ILEP, 3rd Ed., 1986.

Kriel, J. Is Medicine Facing a Philosophical Crisis? *The Medical Observer*, RSA, Sept. 1988, plus and 15.

Languillon, J. Prècis de Léprologie, 2nd Ed. (1986), Masson, Paris.

Lendrum, F.C. The Tragic Name of Leprosy. *Modern Hosp.* 64 (1945): 79–80.

———. The Name Leprosy. *Am.J.Trop.Med. & Hyg.* I (1952): 999–1008.

———. Leprosy. Correspondence, *JAMA* (January 19, 1952): 222.

Lechat, M.F. The Way towards Eradication of Hansen's Disease. Sasakawa Memorial Health Foundation, 2nd Ed., June 1981.

Letayf, S. Recherche sur la Mentalité des Malades de la Lèpre. *Sep. Rev. Psi. Normal e Pathologica* 1 (1955): 3–59.

Levenstein, J.H. Family Medicare, Medical Bureaucracies and Society. *J. South African Academy of Family Practice/Primary Health Care* 9 (1988): 173–182.

Levinsky, N.G. The Doctor's Master. *New Eng. J. Med.* 311 (1984): 1573–1575.

Lichtwardt, H.A. Why Not Change the Name? *The Star*, 1948.

Mallac (de), M.J. Onset and Pattern of Deformity in Leprosy. *Lep. Rev.* 37 (1967): 71–91.

————. Letter to the Editor. *Far East Med. J.* 9 (1971): 108.

McDougall, A.C.M. and Yamalkar, S.J. Leprosy: Basic Information and Management. CIBA-GEIGY, 1987.

Mechanic, D. Public Perception of Medicine. *New Eng. J. Med.* 312 (1985): 181–183.

Medical Man (A): The Stigma of Leprosy—A Personal Experience. *Lep. Rev.* 43 (1972): 83–84.

Meisels-Navon, L. The Paradoxical Stigma of Leprosy. *Int. J. Lep.* 57 (1989); Abstr. Cong. Pprs. FP 225: 348.

Munoz, F.U. and Storkan, M.A. Family Reactions to Leprosy in a Group of Mexican-American Patients. *Int. J. Lep.* 36 (1968); Abstr. Cong. Pprs. XIII 158: 635.

Noordeen, S.K. The Present Status of Leprosy Vaccine Development. *Southeast Asian J. Trop. Med. & Pub. Hlth.* 19 (1988): 525–534.

Oliveira, M.L.W et al. Multi-Media Educational Campaign about Hansen's disease. *Int. J. Lep.* 57 (1989); Abstrc. Cong. Pprs. PO 517: 307.

Ottendorf, T.H.M. and Vries, R.R.P. HLA Class II Immune Response and Suppression Genes in Leprosy. Proc. IV Europ. Lep. Symp. on Lep. Res., Genoa, 1986, Hlth. Coop. Pprs. 7 (1988): 163–177.

Pearson, E.A. Leprosy or Hansen's Disease: A Study of Semantic Conflict. *D. Hans.* 1 (1977), 1: 44–47.

Pre-Congress Workshop. *Leprosy Review* 59 (1988): 284–307.

Rolston, M.A. and Chesteen, H.E. The Identification of Psychological Factors Related to the Rehabilitation of Leprosy Patients. Final Report, August 1970, The School of Social Welfare, Louisiana State University, Baton Rouge.

Rotberg, A. The Serious Latin-American Problems Caused by the Complex "Leprosy": The Word, the Disease and an Appeal for World Co-operation. *Lep. Rev.* 43 (1972): 96–105.

————. The Ancient. Permanent and Powerful Counter-education with the Word "Leprosy" and its Frustration through a New Terminology. Paper presented at the Xth International Leprosy Congress, Bergen, 1973.

————. Letter to the Editor. *Lep. Rev.* 45 (1974): 343–344.

————. Name Changes Reflect Trends. *Int. J. Lep.* 50 (1982): 117–118.

Ryrie, G.A. The Psychology of Leprosy. *Lep. Rev.* 22 (1951): 13–24.

Sankalia, N.S. The Psycho-social Problems of Leprosy Patients in Greater Bombay. *Int. J. Lep.* 36 (1968); Abstrc. Cong. Pprs. XIII 152: 632.

Shanmuganandan, S. et al. Social Aspects of Leprosy: An Analysis of Attitudes and Behaviour of the Patients. *Int. J. Lep.* 57 (1989); Abstrc. Cong. Pprs. PO 326: 361.

Skinsnes Law, A. Challenging the Stigma: From Leprosy to AIDS *Int. J. Lep.* 57 (1989); Abstrc. Cong. Pprs. FP 247:352.

Skinsnes. O.K. and Elvove, R.N. Leprosy in Society V: "Leprosy" in Occidental Literature. *Int. J. Lep.* 38 (1970): 294–306.

Skinsnes. O.K. Leprosy in Society I: "Leprosy Has Appeared on the Face." *Lep. Rev.* 35 (1964): 21–35.

———. Leprosy in Society II: The Pattern of Concept and Reaction to Leprosy in Oriental Antiquity. *Lep. Rev.* 35 (1964): 106–122.

———. Leprosy in Society III: The Relationship of the Social to the Medical Pathology of Leprosy. *Lep. Rev.* 35 (1964): 175–181.

———. Leprosy in Society IV: The Genesis of Lepra-Angst. *Lep. Rev.* 39 (1969): 223–228.

———. Leprosy and the New English Bible. *Int. J. Lep.* 38 (1970): 310–312.

———. Letter to the Editor, *Far East Med. J.* 9 (1971): 307–308.

———. Compilation of Leprosy Equivalent Designations. Editorial, *Int. J. Lep.* 42 (1974): 204–208.

Stigma of Leprosy: Editorial. *Lep. Rev.* 43 (1972): 69–72.

Stringer, T.A. Leprosy and a "Disease Called Leprosy." *Lep. Rev.* 44 (1973): 70–74.

Tas, J. On the Leprosy of the Bible. Proc. 7th Int. Cong. on the History of Science, Jerusalem, August 3, 1953.

Warren, A.G. Are Deformities Stigmatizing? A Surgeon's Approach. *Lep. Rev.* 43 (1972): 74–82.

WHO/RPD/ACHR: Health Research Strategy, Geneva, 1986.

Zhou, D. et al. On Suicide among Leprosy Patients. *China Lep. J.* 2 (1987): 240–243. Author's English Abstract. Current Lit., *Int. J. Lep.* 56 (1988): 489.

The Immunological Dispensation

While one is gratified with a quantum of knowledge mostly attributable to the hardware of the immune response in Hansen's disease, the software orchestrating that response has not been fully elucidated.[1]

That grand old man of Hansen's disease, Kensuke Mitsuda of Japan, was the first one[2] to set up the Mitsuda's Antigen (lepromin) test.[3] Some fourteen years later his countryman, Fumio Hayashi, confirmed the prognostic value of that test, an event that laid down the foundation of all subsequent development of the immunology of the disease as reminded by Lechat (1980). While such a development spells an ongoing process fraught with many unanswered questions still, there is enough evidence by now that:

- Inasmuch as "a good deal is expected still to fit both patients and their lesions in all immune system data generated by in vitro model systems, the revolution occurring in basic immunology, and the onslaught of molecular biology will all combine to make leprosy one of the most researched infectious diseases," as expressed by Mshana and Nilsen (1988).

- Hansen's disease encompasses the entire gradient of the immune response, in the words of Lagrange and Hurtrel (1986). In the view of Harboe (1985), the disease may to a great extent be considered an immunological entity, in that most of its symptoms and important complications are due to reactions against antigenic elements liberated from Hansen's bacillus (*M. leprae*).

- The various forms of the disease developing after infection might well be influenced by genetic factors,[4] hence the significant impetus given to the study of immunogenics for determining the identity and mode of action of those factors, as pointed out by

Ottenhoff and de Vries (1988), mentioning several authors as well. It means that the diverse responses to the antigens liberated from the bacillus determine the disease spectrum in terms of clinicopathological findings via, possibly, HLA-linked genes.

- In established infection by the bacillus, the outcome is most likely determined by the development of cellular immunity, or its failure, as remarked by Bryceson (1981), i.e., the host immune response is responsible for the pathological consequences of Hansen's disease, including the variability in clinical symptomatology of the disease (Mshana and Nilsen, 1986).

- The most important and fundamental immunological issue, apart from that of tolerance, which remains unsolved is the nature of selective unresponsiveness in polar multibacillary (PM) or LL (lepromatous) form as indicated by Bloom (1986) and others, or, as stated elsewhere, Hansen's disease is the "only example in man of specific unresponsiveness liable, with reasonable frequency, to be overcome by immunization and immunotherapy."

- As intimated by Bloom and Mehra (1984), the disease is an unfolding one, "a unique system of probing and intervening to control immunoregulatory mechanisms in man." Otherwise expressed, Hansen's disease offers "the unique opportunity to study the immune mechanisms that might prove a model for other chronic conditions, whether infectious or non-infectious" (Ottenhoff and de Vries, 1988), a view concurring earlier on with that of van den Enden and de Vries (1984).

- The future of epidemiology is tied up with progress in immunology, the latter called upon to provide immunological tools liable to determine, as pointed out by Lechat (1980), both the nature and spread of infection by Hansen's bacillus (*M. leprae*), define groups at risk of developing the polar multibacillary (PM) or LL (lepromatous) form of the disease.

In view of the central role of immunology in Hansen's disease, it would be appropriate to recall in the first place those principles of immunoregulation and the expression of the immune response (IR) to the antigenic elements liberated from the bacillus as prerequisites to the possible sequence of events in the immuno-pathological process.

The Master Immuno-regulators

> More lies in store as to the precise role of those major components of the immune system: lymphocytes, macrophages, and their subsets or phenotypes.

The three components of the immune system, namely, genetical, cellular and molecular, are combined in an extremely complex, sophisticated, yet mutually dependent network, the main function of which being the maintenance of homeostasis[5] and health, as has been indicated. Only the cellular component need be considered here.

The immune system or lymphoid immune system[6] is a unique sequence of events shaped by the nature of antigens,[7] such a system not being under the control of a particular organ but regulated by immune cells, all of which act individually.

Immune cells specifically involved in the immune response comprise:

(i) Two types of lymphocytes[8]: Thymus-dependent or helper-T cells (Th-cells) and B cells originating from bone-marrow via lymph nodes. Both of these populations of cells look similar yet differ in function[9] and communicate with each other by way of lymphokines.[10] As Rosen et al. (1984) remark: "T cells and B cells are generated in different microenvironments, develop as separate lineages, and express different kinds of antigen receptors, but they work together in discriminating between self and non-self." This ability is, incidentally, the crucial distinction since, as well known, failure to do so results in one of the most devastating errors of the immune system: autoimmune diseases. In the context of cell-mediated immunity (CMI), T-cells have a high binding affinity for the antigens of—in this case—Hansen's bacillus (*M. leprae*), in that they are able to "recognize" or "see" those antigens via receptors on the cell membranes,[11] thus allowing them to couple with, or bind to, antigen-presenting macrophages.[12]

(ii) Helper T-cell sub-populations or phenotypes: Th1, Th2, and Th3 defined on the basis of their surface phenotypes, function, and capacity to produce different lymphokines; cytotoxic or "killer" cells; and suppressor cells (Ts cells), all of which are key elements in the chain of events leading to the overcoming of the invading organism.

(iii) Macrophages,[13] which, anatomically close to lymphocytes, play a critical role as an antigen-presenting cell (APC), in that they, too, "recognize" or "see" antigens and act on bacteria by ingesting them into the vacuoles of their cytoplasm, finally digesting them by means of their lysosomal enzymes.[14]

The key role of lymphocytes and macrophages in the immune system is reflected by the dominance of these immune cells in the histology of lesions in Hansen's disease to be fully discussed later on. Thus:

Paucibacillary and borderline groups	Multibacillary form
• Lymphocytes +++ at the periphery	• Lymphocytes virtually absent
• Macrophages (epithelioid cells) at the centre with a few, if any, AFB	• Macrophages (histiocytes not activated into epitheloid cells) loaded with AFB+++

Chain of Events

> The terrain is getting more familiar, but the overall strategy inconclusive still.

The lymphocyte and macrophage-mediated factors and the likely chain of events leading to the killing of Hansen's bacillus (*M. leprae*), or arrest of its multiplication, are outlined below, even though that, as regards the aforesaid killing, no conclusion has been reached yet.

As mostly expounded by Godal (1984),

• upon engulfing the pathogens followed by their intracellular multiplication, macrophages as antigen-presenting cells[15] seize the antigens of Hansen's bacillus (*M. leprae*) and display them on their surface. Only a selected few of the millions of the circulating lymphocytes can reportedly "recognize" or "see" those antigens by coupling with, or binding to, them. This lymphocytic (T-cell)-macrophage interaction is thought of as a mutually and highly sophisticated process not fully understood.

Macrophages, apart from displaying on their surface antigens derived from Hansen's bacillus (*M. leprae*), have also a high concentration of HLA-DR molecules,[16] both of which are required for T-cell activation; so also is interleukin-I (IL-I) produced by antigen-presenting cells.[17] This is the initial response or inductive phase to antigens of the bacillus.

- HLA-DR expression and production of IL-I, probably under control of subset helper T-cell population (Th1), plus macrophages are needed for T-cell activation, i.e., eliciting of a T-cell immune response or generating sensitized T lymphocytes. This is the regulatory phase, or central level of the immune response,[18] characterized by two phenomena: T-cell proliferation and production of interleukin-2 (IL-2), or T-cell growth factor, by a second subset of helper T-cell population (Th2); and receptors for IL-2 produced by a third subset of helper T-cell population (Th3).[19]

- The pace is set for the third and final step of T-cell response to Hansen's bacillus (*M. leprae*), namely the effector phase or T-cell mediated intracellular killing of the bacilli by means of lymphokines endowed with chemotectic properties, or macrophage activating factor (MAF) probably identified with gamma interferon, which activate macrophages to kill and digest the bacilli they have engulfed.[20]

The Immune Response in Hansen's Disease

> "While the immune response is of central importance in the various manifestations of the disease, how soon is it elicited following infection is not known."[21]

The immune response following infection with Hansen's bacillus (*M. leprae*) is a complex one since partly cellular and partly humoral in nature. Only the cellular aspect thereof will be considered here, with the reservation that the immune response (i) covers more than one phenomenon, (ii) is mediated by more than one type of cell and its subset (Maier, 1987), (iii) there is no consensus whether the route of infection controls it, and (iv) whether a gene governs the type of immune response (Demenais and Feingold, 1986), the nature of the genetic component being, moreover, unknown according to Nath (1983). The median view is that, while there is no clear-cut evidence as to the genetic factors playing a really major role in regulating the immune response, the subset or genotype may have some influence on the disease spectrum in the view of Strickland (1985).

There is a considerable body of evidence that the immune response determines the bacterial load of the patient, dictates the modalities of the clinical manifestation of the disease, this bearing equally on the classification of the latter.[22] While the disease, in turn, hinges on the shifting balance between cell-mediated immunity or CMI[23] and humoral immune response[24] to the antigenic elements liberated from Hansen's bacillus (*M. leprae*), the ultimate prognosis will be determined by the capacity of the patient to respond im-munologically to the invading organism, and while the clinical forms of types of the disease are a function of the patient's degree of specific immuno-competence or immuno-incompetence for that matter, the virulence of the bacillus does not come into it.[25]

Inasmuch as the immune response determines both the nature and severity of Hansen's disease according to the resistance or cell-mediated immunity of the host to the bacillus, the immunological characteristics of sub-clinical infection, the time interval between initial infection with the bacillus and appearance of the first clinical signs of the disease come presumably into it, too. So do nerve damage and skin lesions as immune-mediated tissue involvement, and reac-tions as immunological complications as a result of delayed hypersen-sitivity reaction (DHR) to antigens liberated from Hansen's bacillus (*M. leprae*).[26]

Stating that the host-dependent variation in immune status is responsible for the diversity of the clinical appearance of the disease is but part of the picture, in that the factors determining that status have not been fully elucidated yet, i.e., those playing a significant role in triggering the host response to antigens of the bacillus have not been worked out in their entirety. In effect, cellular events underlying the immune response in the disease process are complex and imperfectly understood, we are told, owing probably to a current lack of adequate language and sufficient knowledge to fully explain immunological events in Hansen's disease, in the words of Goihman-Yar (1980), another drawback being that until the bacillus is cultivated in vitro the study of the immune response will be made difficult still, let alone the variability of the pathogen from region to region as has been altogether acknowledged.

Maier (1987) is of opinion that "any conclusion must be tentative because our knowledge about the mechanisms of the immune system, and of T-cells in particular, is not complete." Moreover, in order to understand the immune response, it is important, pursues the author, to discover the various roles all the concerned cells play, individually and in a concerted way.

The Selective Immunological Unresponsiveness State

> The immuno-deficiency to the antigens of Hansen's bacillus (*M. leprae*) in polar multi-bacillary (PM) or LL patients is the major issue of the disease, if not the greatest challenge immunologists are facing at the moment.

Why, as has been asked, does the host system fail to attack Hansen's bacillus (*M. leprae*), or mount an efficient cell-mediated immunity to the bacilli[27] when these are thriving in countless numbers in cells and tissues? Why the immune system is subverted in one individual and not in another, points altogether to a fundamental issue in hansenology (leprology): the immuno-deficiency in polar multi-bacillary (PM) or LL patients,[28] let alone the unanswered time of origin and reversibility attendant to it, as has been pointed out.

The mechanism(s) of this unresponsiveness state,[29] however selective, is foremost to one's understanding of immune tolerance in man, as remarked by Modlin et al. (1986). Earlier on, Bryceson (1982) makes it clear that the defect of cell-mediated immunity in polar multibacillary or LL patients is important in three situations:

(i) The inability of the LL patients to eliminate dead or degraded bacilli, which remain as depots of antigens capable of maintaining immune suppression and eliciting type- and/or immune-complex-mediated reactions or ENL, which may have modulating effects on the immune response; (ii) the defect of cell-mediated immunity allows the multiplication of persistent bacilli in long treated LL patients and so under-lies the phenomenon of relapse and possibly sulphone resistance; (iii) the defect may permit the maintenance of a reservoir of infection in the community in the form of the early diagnosed LL cases.

Harboe (1985) enjoins in saying that:

Detailed understanding of this basic immuno-deficiency in lepromatous leprosy may provide new means for immunotherapy directed against the correction of this defect which would be of utmost importance for the prevention of relapse. Increased knowledge of the nature of this defect and how it is induced is also essential with regard to the development of techniques for prevention of lepromatous leprosy and the efficacy of vaccination procedures.

Several hypotheses have been forwarded to account for the many immunological perturbations in the polar multibacillary (PM) or LL form of Hansen's disease, more particularly the specific T-cell un-responsiveness to antigenic elements liberated from the bacillus, and characterized by the absence of delayed hypersensitivity (DHR), in vitro lymphocytic proliferation and IL-2 and gamma interferon production, as remarked by Ramos et al. (1989):

- Host factors playing admittedly a key role, Rotberg, way back in 1937, postulated a natural or N-factor present in the majority of people and, subsequently, the Hansen Anergic Fringe (HAF) upon the assumption that it affects the minority of the population genetically incapable of developing that variety of specific im-munity to Hansen's bacillus (*M. leprae*) leading to a Mitsuda negative reaction (Rotberg, 1985). In short, the HAF is the hypothetical failure or dysfunction of an immune response gene liable to explain the pathogenesis of the polar multibacillary (PM) or LL form of the disease. For Rotberg (1985), and from an epidemiological standpoint, HAF is (i) the Mitsuda-negative frac-tion of the population who continues as such after infection with the bacillus *M. tuberculosis* or BCG; (ii) the human reservoir that harbors the organism and thus perpetuates the contagiosity in endemic areas.

However, the genetic nature of HAF awaits confirmation

through an appropriate method to identify those persons lacking this factor, in the words of Newell (1966), or, as admitted by Rotberg himself (1985): "The magnitude of HAF cannot be properly assessed until precise quantification thereof be carried out in various endemic and non-endemic areas."

On the other hand, should the above hypothesis be substantiated on genetic grounds, it would prove quite an unpopular one in view of the social implications involved or, as Mshana and Nilsen (1988) observed, would not augur well with current efforts at developing a vaccine specific to Hansen's bacillus (*M. leprae*).

For Chakravarti and Vogel,[30] genetic factors alone are unlikely to be the principal determinants of the immuno-deficiency in polar multibacillary (PM) or LL patients. In the opinion of van den Enden and de Vries (1984), evidence indicates so far that HLA-linked genes do not influence susceptibility to Hansen's disease per se, but rather determine the type of the disease to develop most probably by controlling the disease-specific response, i.e., the HLA-linked control of the susceptibility to polar multibacillary (PM) or LL form of the disease deserves special attention.

Kikuchi et al. (1986) concur with the above view by suggesting the existence of an HLA-linked major gene that controls susceptibility to polar multibacillary (PM) or LL form through T-cell regulation.

Results obtained by Abel et al. (1989) suggest that the gene controlling susceptibility to Hansen's disease might be different from the gene controlling susceptibility to the paucibacillary form of the disease through successive stages of the immune response.

In the final analysis, it is perhaps wise to reflect that "in the presence of the environmental component required for the manifestation of a disease, its frequency is largely determined by genetic constitution. Nevertheless, however prone an individual may be genetically, he is affected only in the appropriate environment. This is as true of non-infectious as of infectious disease."[31]

- Suppressor activity of polar multibacillary (PM) or LL macrophages, abnormal macrophage function with defective presentation of the antigens to the immune system, or defective macrophage function resulting in the capacity to kills Hansen's bacilli (*M. leprae*) envisaged by Mehra et al. in 1982[32] seems to have run out of favor, if not refuted claim,[33] in that lymphocytes from HLA-D of identical siblings responded strongly—even though in vitro—to the bacillus, together with macrophages from polar multibacillary (PM) or LL patients. In a similar context, Nath (1983) observes that, if implicated, defective macrophage function alone could not explain the specific antigen-related unresponsiveness unless mediated through specific T-cells.

Maier (1987) states that, experimentally, "there is no difference in the ability of macrophages from tuberculoid patients as well as from lepromatous patients to digest washed and heat-killed bacilli; no difference either in enzyme contents of these macrophages, while others show the opposite to be true; macrophages from tuberculoid and lepromatous patients seem to be perfectly capable to phagocytize a variety of gram-positive and gram-negative bacteria, and response normally to lymphokines."

- Absolute deficiency in T-cell recognition of the bacillus, or lack of the bacillus responsive helper T-cell, would explain the cell-mediated unresponsiveness in polar multibacillary (PM) or LL patients, as has been advocated.
- Suppression by monocytes and/or their products or suppressor (Ts) cell activity blocking the responsiveness of T-cells to other specific or cross-reactive determinants to Hansen's bacillus (*M. leprae*) was put forward by Mehra et al. (1982), Bloom and Mehra (1984) and van den Enden and de Vries (1984), although—as believed by other authors—the ultimate mechanism relating to Ts cells in preventing helper (Th) T-cells from function is not clear.

Gill and Godal (1987) foresee a defect in T-cell population brought about by suppressor (Ts) cells which have been induced by antigens specific to the bacillus. Mshana and Nilsen (1988) observe that, even though their role in the pathogenesis of polar multibacillary (PM) or LL form is, at best, not clearly understood, Ts cells were likely to be operative therein, on the grounds that (i) PM (LL) patients respond normally to mycobacterial antigens other than those of Hansen's bacillus (*M. leprae*), hence implying a specific response in these patients to the bacillus; (ii) large amount of anti-antibodies of the bacillus in PM (LL) patients point to T-cells that respond to the bacillus and help B cells to produce antibodies; (iii) since in some of these patients exogenous interleukin-2 production was being probably hampered by suppressor

(Ts) cells; (iv) manipulation of the immune system to achieve energy is almost always accompanied by the presence of Ts cells.

- Defect in interleukin-1 (IL-1) production is unclear, but, according to Godal (1984), lack or failure or suppression of IL-2 is, on the other hand, of key importance.[34] In other words, in the view of Longley et al. (1986), the immuno-deficiency in PM (LL) patients is due to a block in the immune cascade at the level of IL-2 receptor expression, the patient's inability to kill the bacilli involving a lack of IL-2 induced T-cell proliferation. Haregewoin (1985) initially observes that the deficient lymphocyte stimulation might be reconstituted by addition of IL-1 to the culture medium. Several other authors find out subsequently that this reconstruction is obtained in some, certainly not all, PM (LL) patients, in fact indicating a heterogenous group probably with different mechanisms triggering cell-mediated immunity, as remarked by Harboe (1988).

- Neither Ts cell activity nor defective IL-2 production, but possibly a low level or lack of Hansen's bacillus (*M. leprae*) responsive cells in the blood circulation of PM (LL) patients is the opinion of Kaplan and Cohn (1987).

- Ferluga et al. (1984) propose that the PM (LL) form of the disease might develop as a result of chronic suppression of specific cellular immunity by anti-idiotypic (Id) antibodies[35] and Id-restricted suppressor lymphocytes, i.e., a potential immuno-tolerizing mechanism.

- A virus-mediated immuno-suppression at the time of infection with Hansen's bacillus (*M. leprae*), or clonal deletion suggested by Strickland (1985) as a possible mechanism, is yet to be confirmed.

- As regards the role of helper T-cell sub-population of genotype, Barnes et al. (1988) think that the relative cell-mediated immune response mounted by PM (LL) patients might be mediated through CD 4 + CDW + memory cells producing gamma interferon. Immunological unresponsiveness state in these patients may reflect the relative absence of this antigen-reactive sub-population or genotype.

- Of late, endogenous glucocorticoid might—albeit subject to confirmation—be involved in the immunological unresponsiveness of the PM (LL) patients by inhibiting IL-2 synthesis, according to Sheriff et al. (1989).

For Convit et al. (1983), there is substantial evidence that the specific immuno-deficiency reaching its maximum in PM (LL) patients is also present in other population groups, including a small portion of the healthy in view of their negative Mitsuda reaction. In the opinion of the authors, that immuno-deficiency might be the case in healthy persons before the onset of clinical disease, i.e., as primary defect.[36]

Earlier on, Stoner (1981) remarks that a primary immuno-deficiency need not be the case; instead, three phases of suppressor mechanism pertaining to the disease spectrum could explain the various types as interplay of suppression and immunity.

It is not clear to Maier (1987) to what extent the specific immuno-deficiency is primary—thus leading to the various types of the disease—or secondary to infection and bacterial load.

It would appear, then, that whether the immuno-deficiency is the result, not the cause, of Hansen's disease itself is an interrogation mark. On the other hand, studies on the mechanisms of antigen-specific unresponsiveness in PM (LL) patients have reportedly been contradictory and difficult to interpret, probably because of the use of heterogenous cell populations in the experiments concerned (Ottenhoff et al., 1986).

Judging by the foregoing, one would tend to agree with Nath (1983) that the mechanism underlying the depression of the host immune response is not elucidated yet; with Bloom and Mehra (1984) that it is unclear in Hansen's disease, or in any other case of clinical unresponsiveness, precisely what factors determine which form of responsiveness will develop; with Ferluga et al. (1984) that reasons for the failure of the immune response in the disease remain obscure and contradictory; with van den Enden and de Vries (1984) that, in essence, specific immuno-deficiency in PM (LL) patients remains an open question.

The Immunological Range of the Disease

> It is no longer possible to envisage Hansen's disease otherwise than mostly the response of the immune system to antigenic elements released from the causative organism.

Hansen's disease has, for many decades, been the cherished province of dermatology and neurology—better still, "the dermatological and neurological duality of that province"—followed more extensively by microbiology, pathology, epidemiology, and, lately, behavioral sciences.

Yet, with the advent of immunology on the scene, it does not mean that that province is being dominated or even taken over by this new discipline. Rather, that immunology has, as the basis of the disease, been there all the time. In other words, owing to the timely intervention and, since then, the increasing interest of immunologists and basic scientists alike in Hansen's disease, it is not a question of perspective anew, but of sheer evidence: the disease turns out to be the most instructive, if not challenging, partition—even though incomplete—of the immunological orchestra.[37]

In fact, for some peculiar reason probably ascribed to tradition and/or conservatism, and in the course of which the obvious has been overlooked—priority in both clinical and didactic practice is still accorded to the effects of Hansen's disease, not to the causes that trigger them off in the first place in terms of immunology.

To put it more succinctly: Shouldn't Hansen's disease, then, be approached from the inside out rather than the other way around as has been hitherto the case? Isn't that what immunology is precisely doing while unfolding the immuno-pathogenesis of the disease in its manifold yet fundamental aspects? On both counts, it avails itself in the affirmative, at least in keeping with the wide range of the present—and future—role played by immunology in the disease process, as shown however summarily in the following chart:

Hansen's bacillus (*M. leprae*)	Immunogenetics	Immunohistology	Immunopathology	Sub-clinical infection
Antigens: Glycolipid antigens(PGL-I, AM-A and B) aimed at testing new drugs, drug resistance, elucidation of mechanisms involved in intracelluar killing of the bacillus **Molecular biology:** Structure and functions of the bacillus which may shed light on how the organism resists killing by the immune system by some individuals **Monoclonal anti-bodies (MAB):** Those specific to the bacillus as a tool for detection of its antigens, rapid diagnosis of the disease and sub-clinical infection, isolation of anti-generical determinants of the organism, viz. anti-MAB in the production of anti-idiotic antibodies as a vaccine substitute	DNA sequencing of the bacillus gene fragments Identification of the comnplete genes and expression of these genes in foreign host micro-organisms with a view to large-scale production of expressed antigens and their application to research on diagnostic tests, immunization, and drug development Mechanism(s) of HLA genes Identification of the bacillus genes involved in protective immunity	The explicit role of predominant T-cell subsets in the production of lymphokines, the relative cell-mediated immunity in polar paucibacillary (PP) or TT patients, and in the immunological unresponsiveness of polar multibacillary (PM) or LL patients	Immunological granuloma as the focal point of the immune response in polar paucibacillary (PP) or TT, paucibacillary borderline (PB) or BT, and borderline (BB) forms of the disease Cell-mediated immunodeficiency in polar multibacillary (PM) or LL form of the disease characterized by a non-immunological or macrophage granuloma.	Immunizing properties

Ongoing and/or prospective studies	Present role of immunology

Pre-clinical infection	Clinical infection	Immunotherapy	Epidemiology	Other research
Time interval between initial infection with Hansen's bacillus and appearance of the first clinical signs of the disease	Forms or types of the disease Classification Prognosis Stability or instability of the disease process Immunoneuropathy and damage to peripheral nerves Skin lesions as morphological expressions of the immune response Immunologically mediated complications or reactions: (i)through delayed hypersensitivity (DHR)(ii) as an immune complex disease	Immunotherapeutic methods Conduct of immunoreactivity trials Immunotherapy combined with chemotherapy	Immunodiagnosis for field use, a priority for the early detection of the disease; identification of high risk groups of people and patients alike; as criterion on which chemotherapy is either instituted or discontinued. immunoprophy—laxis or immunological intervention for the protection of populations at risk by means of vaccination purposes (cf. sub-unit candidate structure, effective vectors for immunization, identification of antigen/epitopes, production of recombinant and/or synthetic candidates, as has been sumitted)	Immunological intact animal models The hansenian as best model More refined techniques and coherent approaches re: (i) probing the cell-mediated immune response (ii) determining the nature of the immune defect in polar multibacillary (PM) or LL patients Mechanism(s) of nerve damage Prediction of immunologically mediated reactions and relapse

in Hansen's disease

Under evaluation and/or foreseen

Notes

1. In other words, as Nath (1983) intimates: "No consensus has been reached as to the central mechanism that would coherently unify the diverse immunological and clinical phenomena seen in the leprosy spectrum in general and lepromatous leprosy in particular."
2. In 1919.
3. Also known as the (early) Fernandez and the (late) Mitsuda reaction.
4. The credit goes to Prof. A. Rotberg for being the first one to draw attention to it as early as 1937, a credit unfortunately not duly acknowledged outside South America.
5. I.e., the tendency to uniformity or stability in the normal body state of the organism (cf. Dorland's Med. Dict.).
6. Or immunity or defense reaction of the human body of which it has been said that it is "one of nature's most incredible and complete creations . . . with a phenomenal ability for dealing with information, for learning and memory, for creating and storing and using information."
7. I.e., alien or foreign substance or immunogen. In the case of Hansen's bacillus (*M. leprae*), for instance, its antigens are marker proteins, a part of the bacillus identity.
8. Lymphocytes are small, actively mobile, non-phagocytic corpuscles, a much larger pool of which being found in the lymph tissue (spleen, bone marrow, lymph nodes, etc.). Both T and B cells are derived from precursor cells in bone marrow, as remarked by Strober and McDevitt (1984). Moreover, in the case of T-cells, the "precursor cells migrate to the thymus, where they develop some of the functional and cell surface characteristics of mature T-cells. Thereafter, the cells migrate to the T-dependent areas of the peripheral lymphoid tissues (paracortical areas of lymph nodes and periarteriolar sheath of the spleen) and enter the pool of long-lived lymphocytes that reticulate from the blood of the lymph."

    Goihman-Yar estimates that effector lymphocyte populations are being subdivided and more, with the result that the exact pairing of lymphocyte receptors, lymphocyte types, and lymphocyte function in man have not been achieved yet. Bloom and Mehra (1984) point out, in turn, that little information is at hand at present, and the requirements for development and amplification of T-cells in any system for that matter. In other words, as Mitchison (1986) indicates, the full potential reservoir of T-cells has not been determined yet.
9. A distinction made only in the early sixties, as has been remarked.
10. I.e., the non-antibody-soluble mediators of cellular immunity according to Holborrow and Lessof (1981), or protein substances playing a leading role in the final overcoming of the invading organism, or chemical signals with a bewildering array of names and function as has been stated, those having been discovered so far being the reported top of the iceberg.
11. Others being B cells, monocytes, and Langhans' giant cells.
12. While Godal (1984) reminds us that T-cell–APC interaction—thought to be a mutually dependent and highly sophisticated process—is not fully understood yet, Draper (1986) queries in the same vein both incidence and nature of the process.
13. Or dendritic cells, which, discovered by Metchnikoff in the 1880s, are

mononuclear cells originating from the hematopoietic system via monocytes and reticulo-endothelial system.

14. It has been suggested that effective macrophage activation to enable mycobacterial destruction is the most important part of the immune response in Hansen's disease, a point of view shared by Goihman-Yar (1980) to the effect that the fate of the bacillus and of the patient is decided inside the macrophage. Unfortunately, one would like to add, unless the cell-mediated immunity is high enough or the macrophage activated by the host immune system against the bacillus, destruction of the invading organism by lysosomal enzymes does not take place as has been advocated.

    Lagrange and Hurtrel (1986) remark that macrophage activation is specific in its induction but non-specific in its expression since it is locally able to inhibit growth and dissemination of other obligate unrelated intracellular multiplying microorganisms. On the other hand, consider macrophage activation by T-cells through lymphokines, of which, according to Mitchison (1986), the principal and clearly identified one is gamma interferon, there being, besides, indicators of other macrophage activating factors (MAFs), i.e., lymphokines and other unidentified proteins, secreted by T-cells. In this context, it is interesting to note that, in the opinion of Bharadwaj, et al. (1987), macrophage activation occurs in polar paucibacillary (PP) or TT patients while passive in PM (LL) patients and immunological complications or reactional states of the disease through a loss of lysosomal function. In short, macrophages maintain their lysosomal morphology in PP (TT) form of the disease, borderline paucibacillary (BP) or BT form, and Jopling's type I reaction associated with the latter, but lose their cellular morphology and cell membrane integrity in PM (LL) form, borderline multibacillary (BM), or BL and Jopling's type II reaction associated with it.

    As to next, the actual killing of Hansen's bacillus (*M. leprae*), Lagrange and Hurtrel (1986) wonder which functional subset of macrophages are involved in the process, and Strickland (1987) queries the variety of microbicidal mechanisms involved in the same process, even less being known about it in the macrophages themselves.

15. Exactly how and at what point in time this presentation occurs after entry of the bacillus in the human body is not known.

16. Or major human histocompatibility complex molecules, actually glycoproteins floating in the plasma membrane of most nuclear cells and involved in the etiology and pathogenesis of many other diseases.

17. In this case, a molecular mediator that, produced by activated T-cells (lymphocytes), is absolutely necessary for the continued proliferation of T-cells.

18. Possibly also, according to Godal (1984), the suppressor circuit, since T-cells are controlled by suppressor (Ts) cells, which may interfere with T-cell activation by blocking IL-2 production as well as production of IL-1 receptors.

19. Actually, Godal (1984) is of the opinion that Th_1, Th_2, and Th_3 may be largely overlapping populations.

20. With two reservations at this juncture: (i) lymphokine activation is acknowledged as being an important mechanism of macrophage activation as already intimated, but whether that mechanism is effective inside Schwann cells is queried by Harboe (1985); (ii) there is no consensus of opinion as regards the role of cytotoxic cells as observed by Mitchison (1986).

21. Harboe, 1985.

22. Bryceson, 1976.

23. Cell-mediated immunity or CMI is a term understood to encompass not only protective immune function but also delayed hypersensitivity (DHR) to antigenic elements liberated from Hansen's bacillus (*M. leprae*) in this case, as well as other cell-mediated reactions known to the immunologist, as has been stated. In Hansen's disease CMI, governed by T-cell–macrophage interaction, determines the position of the host on the disease spectrum.
24. Or antibody-mediated hypersensitivity. In this respect, antibodies do not seem to play a protective role in Hansen's disease since, as has been pointed out, they are unable to get intracellularly at the bacillus.
25. Or, as Bryceson (1982) puts it: "For the clinician, the importance of the immune response is those aspects thereof which determine (i) the type of the disease the patient develops, (ii) the clinical features of the disease at that point of the spectrum, (iii) the stability or instability of his disease, (iv) the complications he may encounter in terms of movement across the spectrum, and reactions, (v) the type of treatment he will need, and its duration, and the prognosis."
26. Delayed hypersensitivity (DHR) to Hansen's bacillus (*M. leprae*) and its antigens, while representing the body's effort to destroy it, correlates with cell-mediated immunity. DHR is measured in vitro by the early Fernandez (24–72 hours) or the late Mitsuda (3–4 weeks) in vivo by the lymphocyte migration inhibitory test (MIF). Skin tests have no diagnostic value, yet a bearing on the prognosis of the disease has been indicated.
27. As made evident by the tests cited above.
28. Immuno-deficiency is a specific cellular form not unique in Hansen's disease, as Harboe (1985) intimates, but is seen in chronic diseases with microorganisms within macrophages.
29. Which, incidentally, persists after prolonged chemotherapy, thus likely to be responsible for relapse, quite a serious problem when it involves PM (LL) patients.
30. Quoted by Bloom and Mehra (1984).
31. WHO Advisory Committee on Health Research, Geneva, 1986.
32. Quoted by Strickland (1985).
33. Stoner et al. (quoted by Harboe, 1985); van den Enden and de Vries (1984); Mahadevan et al. (1985).
34. I.e., the amount of which possibly determining the balance between immunity and unresponsiveness.
35. I.e., self-antigenic epitopes located on lymphocyte receptors and antibody molecules.
36. I.e., a primary malfunction or physical absence of some components of cell-mediated immunity (Strickland, 1985).
37. "Endocrinologists speak of an endocrine orchestra, implying an interaction between the various components of the system which determines overall endocrine function. This idea might well be adapted by immunologists" (*The Lancet*, leading article, January 27, 1968).

References

Abel, L. et al.: Genetic Susceptibility to Leprosy on a Caribbean Island: Linkage Analysis with Fire Markers. *Int. J. Lep.* 57 (1989):465–471.

Barnes, P.F. et al.: A comparative study of the immunohistology of leprosy and tuberculosis. *Int. J. Lep.* 56 (1988): 688–689.

Bharadwaj, V.P. et al.: Ultracytochemical Studies of Lysosomal Function in the Macrophages of Human Leprosy (I). *Int. J. Lep.* 55 (1987): 328–332.

Bloom, B.R. Towards a Leprosy Vaccine. *World Health.* May 1985: 3–5.

———. Learning from Leprosy: a Perspective on Immunology and the Third World. *J. Imm.* 137 (1986), 1: I–X.

Bloom, B.R. and Mehra, V. Immunological Unresponsiveness in Leprosy. *Imm. Rev.* 80 (1984): 5–28.

Bryceson, A.D.M. Immunology of Leprosy. *Lep. Rev.* 47 (1976): 235–243.

———. Immunology. Europ. Lep. Symp. Genoa, May 1981, Hlth. Coop. Pprs. 1 (1982): 35–38.

———. Summary of Europ. Lep. Symp. Genoa, May 1981, Hlth. Coop. Pprs. 1 (1982): 183–184.

Convit, J. et al. Immunotherapy and Immunoprophylaxis in Leprosy. *Lep. Rev.* 54 (1983), Spc. Issue: S75–S95.

Demenais, F. and Feingold, N. HLA and Leprosy. Authors' Summary. Current Lit., *Int. J. Lep.* 54 (1986): 691.

Draper, P. Structure of *Mycobacterium leprae. Lep. Rev.* 57 (1986), Supp. 2: 15–20.

Ferluga, V. et al. Hypothesis: Possible idiotypic suppression of cell-mediated immunity in lepromatous leprosy. *Lep. Rev.* 55 (1987): 221–227.

Fleury, R. and Bacchi, C.E. S-100 Protein and Immunoperoxidase Technique as an Acid in the Histopathological Diagnosis of Leprosy. *Int. J. Lep.* 55 (1987): 338–344.

Gill, H.D. and Godal, T. Deficiency of Cell-mediated Immunity in Leprosy. Authors' Summary. Current Lit., *Int. J. Lep.* 55 (1987):177.

Goihman-Yar, M. Thoughts on the Immunology of Leprosy. *Int. J. Lep.* 48 (198?): 435–439.

Godal, T. Leprosy Immunology—Some Aspects of the Role of the Immune System in the Pathogenesis of Disease. *Lep. Rev.* 55 (1984): 407–414.

Harboe, M. The Immunology of Leprosy. In *Leprosy*, Ed. R.C. Hastings, Churchill Livingstone, 1985, 53–87.

Haregewoin, A. Investigation into T-cell Function in Leprosy with Special Emphasis on the Immunological Unresponsiveness of Lepromatous Leprosy. A.H.R.I., Addis Ababa, Lab. for Immunological Research, Norsk Hydro's Institute for Cancer Research, Oslo, 1985.

Holborrow, J. and Lessof, M. Immuno Mechanism in Health and Disease. *Immunology,* Med. Int., August 1981, 213–218.

Kaplan, G. and Cohn, Z.A. The Immunobiology of Leprosy. Author's Summary. *Int. J. Lep.* 55 (1987): 177–178.

Kikuchi, I. et al. An HLA-linked Gene Controls Susceptibility to Lepromatous Leprosy through T-cell Regulation. *Lep. Rev.* 57 (1986), Supp. 2: 139–142.

Langrange, P.H. and Hurtrel, B. Induction of Protective Immunity to Mycobacterial Infection. *Lep. Rev.* 57 (1986), Supp. 2: 231–244.

Lechat, M.F. The Way towards Eradication of Hansen's Disease. Sasakawa Memorial Health Foundation, September 1980, 1–14.

Longley, B.J. et al. Lepromin Stimulates Interleukin-2 Production and Interleukin-2 Receptor Expression in situ in Lepromatous Leprosy Patients. *Lep. Rev.* 57 (1986): 189–190.

Maier, M. The Relation between Allergy and Immunity in Leprosy. *Int. J. Lep.* 55 (1987): 116–139.

Mitchison, N.S. The Lessons to Take Home *Lep. Rev.* 57 (1986): 305–308.

Modlin, R.L. et al. T-lymphocyte clones from leprosy skin lesions. *Lep. Rev.* 57 (1986): 143–147.

Mshana, R.N. and Nilsen, R. Leprosy: The Immunologist and the Patient. Editorial, *Int. J. Lep.* 56 (1988): 314–322.

Narayanan, R.B. Immunopathology of Leprosy Granulomas—current status—a revision. *Lep. Rev.* 59 (1988): 75–82.

Nath, I. Immunology of Human Leprosy—Current Status. *Lep. Rev.* 31 (1986), Spec. Issue: S31–S41.

Newell, H.K. An Epidemiologist View of Leprosy. *Bull. WHO* 34 (1966): 827–857.

Ottenhoff, T.H.M. and de Vries, R.R.P. HLA Class II Immune Response and Suppression Genes in Leprosy. Europ. Lep. Symp., Genoa, May 1981, Hlth. Coop. Pprs. 1 (1982): 163–177.

Ramos, Theresa et al. T-Helper Cell Sub-populations and the Immune Spectrum of Leprosy. *Int. J. Lep.* 57 (1989): 73–81.

Rosen, F.S. et al. The Primary Immuno-deficiencies (I). *New England J. Med.* 311 (1984): 235–240.

Rotberg, A. Some Aspects of Immunity in Leprosy and their Importance in Epidemiology, Pathogenesis and Classification of Forms—Based on 1529 Lepromin Tested Cases. *Sep. Rev. Braz. Leprologia* V (1937), Numero Special: 45–95.

———. The Hansen Anergic Fringe. *Acta Lepr.* IV (1985), 3: 347–354.

Sheriff, S. et al. Glucocorticoid Receptor and Lymphocytes in Leprosy. *Int. J. Lep.* 57 (1989); Abstr. Cong. Pprs. FP 049: 313.

Stoner, G.L. Hypothesis: Do Phases of Immuno-suppression During a *M. leprae* Infection Determine the Leprosy Spectrum? *Lep. Rev.* 52 (1981): 1–10.

Strickland, N.H. The Influence of Immuno-suppression and Immuno-deficiency on Infection with Leprosy and Tuberculosis. *Int. J. Lep.* 53 (1985): 86–99.

Strober, A. and McDevitt, H.O. Immunologic Disorders. *Current Med. Diagnosis and Treatment* (1984): 1066–1083.

Van den Enden, W. and de Vries, R.R.P. Occasional Review—HLA and Leprosy: a Re-evaluation. *Lep. Rev.* 55 (1984): 89–104.

Van Voorhis, W.C. et al. The Cutaneous Infiltrates of Leprosy. *New England J. Med.* 307 (1982): 1593–1597.

WHO/RPD/ACHR/86: Health Research Strategy, Advisory Committee on Health Research, WHO, Geneva 1986.

The Crux of the Matter

<blockquote>

The immune-mediated tissue involvement in Hansen's disease is not fully understood, even reportedly poorly so. Thus, any unifying approach to the problem is, from the outset, bound to be a tentative one.

</blockquote>

The immuno-pathological process encompassing incipient infection by Hansen's bacillus (*M. leprae*) and overt manifestation of the disease rests on a multifactorial contingency or fortuitous circumstances, as has been intimated. In fact, the disease process involves a series of events neither completely understood nor altogether known, like, for instance, the possible influence of the portal of entry of the bacillus, how soon the immune response is set in motion following initial infection, the infective load, and behavior of the bacillus, as remarked by Harboe (1985).

In view of the latency or long incubation period of Hansen's disease, it would seem that there is a critical phase following infection that predicts the future position of the patient on the disease spectrum, as has been suggested, even though, as pointed out by Bloom and Mehra (1984), it is unclear what determines whether the infection will be contained or will develop towards PM (LL) forms of the disease or PP (TT) form.

What is needed is neither a master blueprint nor a linear model, but a conceptual framework purporting to the possible sequence of events the moment Hansen's bacillus (*M. leprae*) gets into the body, right down to the ultimate fate shared by the various clinical forms or types of the disease: immune-mediated tissue involvement in terms of nerve damage and skin lesions mostly.

To this effect—even though subject to modification—the underlying diagram illustrates the point sequentially as follows:

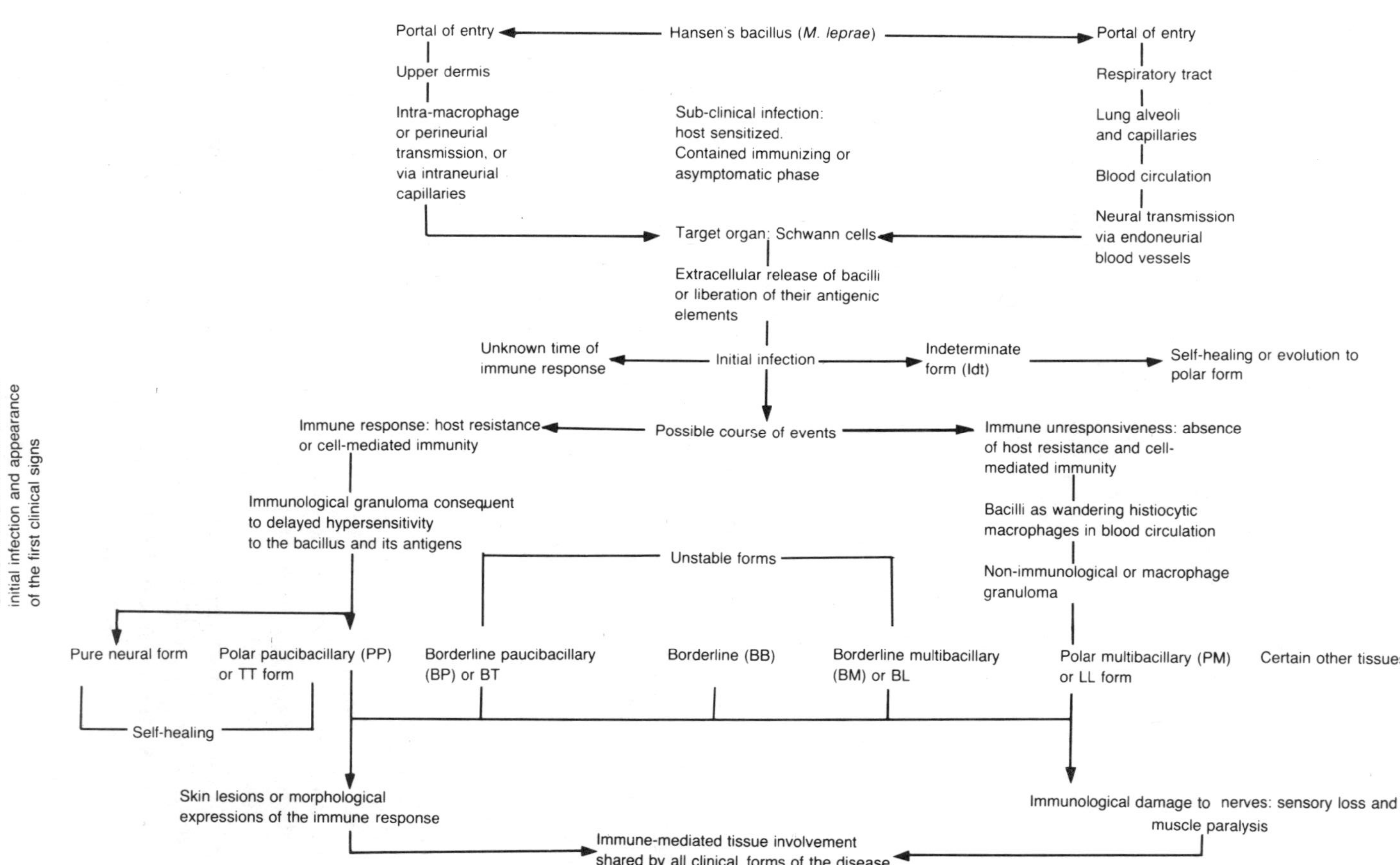

Hansen's bacillus (M. leprae)
Portal of entry
Upper dermis
Intra-macrophage or perineurial transmission, or via intraneurial capillaries
Sub-clinical infection: host sensitized. Contained immunizing or asymptomatic phase
Portal of entry
Respiratory tract
Lung alveoli and capillaries
Blood circulation
Neural transmission via endoneurial blood vessels
Target organ: Schwann cells
Extracellular release of bacilli or liberation of their antigenic elements
Unknown time of immune response
Initial infection
Indeterminate form (Idt)
Self-healing or evolution to polar form
Immune response: host resistance or cell-mediated immunity
Possible course of events
Immune unresponsiveness: absence of host resistance and cell-mediated immunity
Immunological granuloma consequent to delayed hypersensitivity to the bacillus and its antigens
Bacilli as wandering histiocytic macrophages in blood circulation
Non-immunological or macrophage granuloma
Unstable forms
Unknown time interval between initial infection and appearance of the first clinical signs
Pure neural form
Polar paucibacillary (PP) or TT form
Borderline paucibacillary (BP) or BT
Borderline (BB)
Borderline multibacillary (BM) or BL
Polar multibacillary (PM) or LL form
Certain other tissues
Self-healing
Skin lesions or morphological expressions of the immune response
Immunological damage to nerves: sensory loss and muscle paralysis
Immune-mediated tissue involvement shared by all clinical forms of the disease.

- Hansen's bacillus (*M. leprae*) as the elusive bacterium.
- Portal of entry of the invading organism as the inconclusive initial inoculum.
- Sub-clinical infection as the most common outcome of exposure to the invading organism.
- Schwann cells as the target organ of Hansen's bacillus (*M. leprae*) through neural transmission from either route: skin or respiratory tract or both.
- Progression to clinical stage when the bacillus is released extracellularly or antigenic elements thereof liberated.
- Initial infection bearing on two unknown factors: (i) the time of onset of the immune response and (ii) the time interval between it and appearance of the first clinical signs of the disease.
- The possible course of events from then on includes the indeterminate (Idt) form of the disease, although it does not belong immunologically to the disease spectrum.
- The subsequent elaboration of the two polar forms of the disease via their immunological focal points, i.e., the immunological granuloma and the non-immunological or macrophage granuloma respectively, with the borderline group in between as the unstable forms.
- The final outcome, as expected, is the common fate shared by the clinical types of Hansen's disease: immune-mediated tissue involvement, of which nerve damage is foremost.

The Elusive Bacterium

> As one of the oldest pathogens known to man—and to which most people are immune—Hansen's bacillus (*M. leprae*) is holding its own in a way hardly comparable to any other bacterium.

What of an antigenically complex causative organism which—the first identified bacterial pathogen in man,[1] the only species of Mycobacteria to invade peripheral nerve, is an obligate intracellular etiological agent invested with a low immuno-pathogenicity,[2] does not satisfy Koch's postulate,[3] and, hence, proves a major impediment to research for more than a century?

A mobile, non spore-forming and gram-positive AFB[4] with strains said to vary from region to region,[5] its pathogenic pedigree, however impressive, is not restricted to *Homo sapiens*: naturally acquired or indigenous Hansen's disease has been found in the chimpanzee (1977), both the mangabey and green African monkeys (1979), while adding up to the score started experimentally by Kirscheim and Storrs in 1975 with the nine-banded armadillo (Dasypus novemcinctus), as a living medium for the production of the bacilli.

A slender, polymorphous rod measuring 0.5 to 2.8 micron[6] with reported minimum infective doses from 40 to 3 solidly staining rods, Hansen's bacillus (*M. leprae*) is found either singly or in masses (globi), the granular, non-solid form of which is degenerate, non-viable.

As intimated by Ridley and Job (1985), the commonest protection site of the bacillus in early lesions is the nerve bundle, the second most common site the sub-epidermis zone just below the basal layer, and an almost equal evidence of the disease.

Barring some viruses, Hansen's bacillus (*M. leprae*) is said to exhibit a unique affinity for peripheral nerves, whereas it is by now accepted that it is rather Schwann cells which act as its protected sites or immunological barriers.

The main characteristics of the bacillus are compounded of (i) an almost avirulence, (ii) a slow cellular growth or generation time,[7] (iii) a low optimal temperature, and (iv) sparing vital organs that confers Hansen's disease its non-fatal chronicity, as has been altogether reported.

Yet, in the view of Stoner (1981), it is the same bacillus that:

> In its flight for survival, employs an escape route: its ability to penetrate and grow in non-defensive cells like Schwann cells, smooth, endothelial cells, smooth muscle-fibre cells which cannot be activated by immunological mechanisms to destroy the invader.

Whether Hansen's bacillus (*M. leprae*) may be a microbe-dependent microorganism in a unique way is debatable;[8] what at this stage is pertinent is that (i) a good deal depends still on the knowledge relating to its antigenic components,[9] molecular and genetical properties, and

(ii) the inability to cultivate it in vitro is hampered by limited under-standing of the organism's biochemical and metabolic processes, as stated by Rees (1985).

No doubt, the determination of the full characteristics and capabilities of the bacillus would:

- Speed up the process of its cultivation on artificial media.
- Sort out its role in the immune response.
- Elucidate the reason(s) for its location in the protected sites.
- Reveal its relatedness or divergence among other strains isolated from patients in different parts of the world.
- Indicate the source of its energy for its survival and proliferation, as has been altogether postulated.
- Allow the complete identification of its antigenic components other than, so far, PGL-1, LAM-A and LAM-B, other protein antigens since, as expressed by Young (1988), the study of those antigens could be a key to understanding immunity in Hansen's disease.
- Lead to development and assessment of more suitable drugs and their derivatives at least able to penetrate the bacterial cell, as intimated by Draper (1986).

The Inconclusive Initial Inoculum

> Mode of entry of Hansen's bacillus (*M. leprae*) might prove a determinant in the development of the disease spectrum.

Inasmuch as the major exit routes of Hansen's bacillus (*M. leprae*) are well known (cf. nose, mouth, and occasionally ulcerated skin lesions on account of their bacillary load in untreated patients, as has been said), site(s) of initial inoculum of the pathogen or its mechanism of transmission remains conjectural, if not unproven, in that views or beliefs about it vary widely, as concurred with by Noordeen (1985).

Intradermal inoculation or epidermal route as mode of entry of the organism is assumed by many past and present authors.[10] In this respect, while it is thought that

- no bacillus is ever found in the intact skin of PP (TT) patients, and very rarely so in the skin lesions of this form of disease,
- and bacilli are equally rare in the intact skin of PM (LL) patients because the highly bacilliferous non-immunological macrophage granuloma in the dermis is separated from the basal layer of the epidermis by a granuloma-free zone.

Job[11] reports that, experimentally, Hansen's bacillus (*M. leprae*) can penetrate the epidermis of unbroken skin of nude mice, especially through hair follicles and sebaceous glands. For the author (1988), there is convincing evidence that entry of the organism occurs at the site of the primary skin lesion.

For Mathur et al. (1989), "if bacillus enters through epidermal route where it is exposed to skin-associated lymphoid tissue (SALT), it probably generates sensitization and can end up either in no disease or tuberculoid spectrum."

On the other hand, many other authors favor the nasal mucosa as the dominant entry site,[12] i.e., through the anterior end of the inferior nasal turbinate, as has been suggested. The possibility of transmission by inhalation appears to be prevailing, in that bacilli are reportedly found in the nasal discharge, a high proportion of which being morphologically intact; their ability to survive for hours or days outside the host is argued by Noordeen (1985). The author also mentions that, experimentally, Rees and McDougall in 1977 succeeded in transmitting the infection to immune-suppressed mice through aerosol containing Hansen's bacillus (*M. leprae*).

It has been postulated that PM (LL) form of the disease results when the bacillus enters the body through the nasal mucosa, an attractive enough possibility yet awaiting confirmation in humans. For Job (1988), both skin and nasal mucosa have, in experimental Hansen's disease, triggered PM (LL) form or borderline multibacillary (BM) or BL form, while PP (TT) form has never been produced in animal models.

Since both skin and respiratory tracts as modes of entry of the bacillus are not fully established yet, Reich (1988) proposes that the organism, having evolved a highly efficient state of parasitism in stable types of populations, the majority of them incubating sub-clinical infection at various levels, it follows that clinical Hansen's disease arises from within the pool of that infection in endemic populations rather than by transmission.

At this stage, appropriate research might shed light on that confounding issue, and its corollaries: transmission of the bacillus and whether mode of entry or route of infection is crucial in the development of the type of the disease spectrum or not, in the view of many authors.

However, for the immediate purpose of this section, should the skin be the portal of entry of Hansen's bacillus (*M. leprae*), it implies that the organism is, as a first step, taken up by the histiocytic macrophage of the skin, penetrating next both sensory and autonomic terminal nerve endings or twigs that are most dense around the pilo-sebaceous complex, and their small blood vessels, then reaching their final destination: Schwann cells. Three other possibilities of bacillary entry are discussed later on in the text.

If the naso-pharynx is the mode of entry of the organism, pathways to the peripheral nerves are via pulmonary alveoli, lung capillaries, blood circulation, and, finally, endoneurial blood vessels as neural transmitters of the organism to Schwann cells.

With skin or respiratory tract as portal of entry of Hansen's bacillus (*M. leprae*), the next consideration is the sensitized host, or sub-clinical infection.

The Sensitized Host

> Sub-clinical infection is the most common outcome of exposure to Hansen's bacillus (*M. leprae*), hence a major link in the control of the disease.

Sensitization of the host by Hansen's bacillus (*M. leprae*), probably in more than 90% of people infected by the organism as has been indicated, implies that the pathogen is eliminated before it is able to reach the Schwann cells, or that the host immune response is good, and apt to detect or destroy bacilli before their multiplication has set in, as intimated by Ridley (1985).

Sub-clinical infection is the symptomless phase of the disease, meaning that the organism, in other words, causes a sub-clinical immunizing infection, but people with delayed or deficient resistance develop Hansen's disease.

Another preferred version is that exposure to Hansen's bacillus (*M. leprae*), although necessary, is not a sufficient etiological component contracting the disease, as the great majority of people exposed to it may become infected without developing any signs or symptoms. Either way, symptomless infected people might, in the view of many authors, provide the essential link in the transmission of the disease.

From an epidemiological standpoint, sub-clinical infection constitutes, as acknowledged, the hidden spread of the disease, hence the great importance of detecting that sort of infection by way of appropriate immuno-diagnostic tools and, by the same token, knowing about the occurrence and pattern of that spread in endemic and partially endemic areas.

The Target Organ

> Despite their key role in the pathogenesis of Hansen's disease, Schwann cells cannot be activated by the immune system to destroy the invading organism.

Schwann cells, derived from monocytes of the blood via non-nuclear cells, are, unlike other phagocytic macrophages, "non-professional cells," as remarked by Ridley and Job (1985), because of their being not well adapted for antigen-presentation. In other words, Schwann cells have no lysosomes, are bounded by basement membranes, and retain antigen as their life-span extends not to weeks, but to years, as has been reported.

Whether Hansen's bacillus (*M. leprae*) shows a special affinity for Schwann cells is by now questionable, as has been intimated: the more acceptable view is that these cells act as host cells to the bacillus (Boddingius, 1981), or as immunologically protected sites of choice, according to Ridley and Job (1985).

Schwann cells are said to be responsible for making myelin in the peripheral nerve, the presence of the bacillus not causing gross structural abnormalities in the myelin sheath (Samuel et al. 1986). As regards the relation of Schwann cells to the immune system, particularly their ill-adapted capacity as antigen-presenting cells (APCs), evidence suggests, in the view of the authors, the possibility for Schwann cells to present foreign antigens to T-cells during nerve infection and thus initiate immune response against the invading organism. The more conservative view of Harboe (1985) is that little is known about the behavior of Schwann cells in relation to the immune system, hence the need for a better understanding of, or insight into, the physiology of these cells, and the early events following infection of Hansen's bacillus (*M. leprae*).

Once infection sets in—by way of skin or respiratory tract—it is less frequently along the axon or neuron[13] that is ensheathed by Schwann cells. More often than not, the first step in the inception of a skin lesion is acknowledged through the presence of the bacillus in a nerve bundle in the skin, i.e., via its normal habitat: Schwann cells.

Having engulfed a practically non-virulent bacillus endowed, moreover, with a long generation time[14] and which it is unable to destroy outright, the Schwann cell favors its growth instead in a limited way through a stage of intra-macrophage infection bound to be consequently a slow one, frequently, if not always so, in the superficial peripheral nerves peculiar to Hansen's disease, i.e., where, as protective and important sites, they are most cool and subject to trauma, as has been said.

The mechanism by which Hansen's bacillus (*M. leprae*) and/or its antigens escape from Schwann cells is a matter of conjecture at this stage; it is probably by a slow leak out of the basal lamina of the cells. This extra-cellular release is presumably the start of initial infection, as has been intimated, but what moment in time the immune response comes into play is not known. One can infer that, depending on the position of the host along the disease spectrum, there is a critical threshold between that initial infection and appearance of the first clinical signs of the disease.

Clinical Spectrum

No other mycobacterial infection encompasses so much on the immune spectrum, comprises such immunological entity as Hansen's disease.

Hansen's disease, acknowledged as being to a great extent an immunological entity, is hence explained by the evidence that its clinical symptomatology and variability are mostly due to reactions against antigenic elements liberated from the bacillus, as already intimated.

The diagram opposite—a modified version of the Ridley Jopling scale[15]—serves the purpose of overview of the various forms or types of the disease to be elaborated next.

The Non-definite Form

The concept of indeterminate (Idt) form of Hansen's disease is a fairly recent one, and its status somehow controversial.[16]

The indeterminate form of Hansen's disease does not fit into its immunological spectrum because in this form immunity is not strong enough and hypersensitivity to the antigenic elements liberated from the bacillus not developed, hence the clinical features that are symptomless, transitory, or inconclusive.[17]

Indeterminate form of the disease is the acknowledged earliest and most macular type, yet not its initial involvement, as believed in some quarters.[18] Found mostly in children and young adults, Idt involves usually a single or a few hypochromic skin lesions, hence—in the absence of immunity—the mild, non-specific response typically described as scattered histiocytes and a lymphocytic reaction around skin appendages.[19] There is no granuloma formation unless evolution towards the PP (TT) form is the case, or even towards the PM (LL) form.

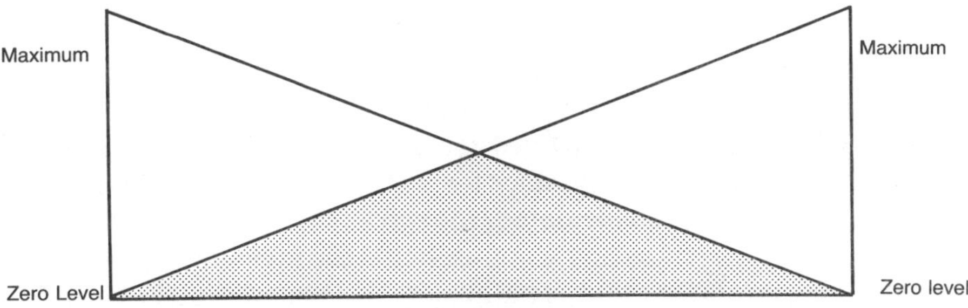

PM or LL

- Immunologically stable end of the spectrum
- Unresponsiveness to antigenic components liberated by the bacillus
- No cell-mediated immunity (CMI)
- Negative Mitsuda reaction
- Maximal bacillary load with globi
- Non-immunological or macrophage granuloma
- Mild to moderate to severe nerve damage as a late phenomenon
- Severe skin lesions (multiple and symmetrical)

BM or BL

- Unstable form
- Negative Mitsuda reaction
- Numerous AFBs, but globi unusual
- Non-immunological or macrophage granuloma with more lymphocytes
- Moderate to severe nerve damage
- Severe skin lesions

BB

- Unstable centre of the spectrum
- Negative Mitsuda reaction
- AFBs moderate in lesions
- Immunological granuloma not focalized into a tubercle
- Moderate to severe nerve damage
- Moderate skin lesions
- Tendency to acute immunological complications or reactions of Type I due to delayed hypersensitivity (DHR)

PP or TT

- Immunologically stable end of the spectrum
- High resistance or cell-mediated immunity (CMI)
- Positive Mitsuda reaction
- Zero bacillary load or growth
- Immunological granuloma focalized into tubercle
- Mild to moderate nerve damage as an early phenomenon
- Mild skin lesions (single or few, asymmetrical)

BP or BT

- Unstable form
- Weakly or moderate postive Mitsuda reaction
- Scanty or rare AFBs
- Immunological granuloma focalized into tubercle
- Peak of acute nerve damage in the course of immunological complications of type I
- Mild to moderate skin lesions.

According to Ridley (1985), after a thorough search of several serial sections, AFB, singly or in small clumps, may be discovered. Mast cells were reported by Liu Tze-Chun et al. (1982) to be far more numerous in Idt than in any other form of the disease, the significance of which has not been elucidated, though.

The immune status being non-definite, the invading organism not established, it follows that the pathogen does not multiply to the point at which it becomes immunologically detectable, as has been remarked, as also the Mitsuda reaction, positive to a various degree or negative yet showing a reciprocal conversion.

One is reminded by Harboe (1985) that although the established clinical and histological picture appears homogenous, the host shows either no immune response to the bacillus or a very weak one. On the other hand, some cases of Idt display an immunity even higher than PP (LL) or PP (TT) form but cannot, in the view of Ridley and Job (1985), be identified.

Owing to the inherent difficulty in diagnosing Idt, and the fact that this form of the disease is reportedly inconclusive but in about half of the cases, the evidence for it calls for, more often than not, the expertise of both dermatologist and histopathologist, as has been recommended. Besides, it is acknowledged that a great number of patients with the indeterminate (Idt) form of Hansen's disease—the evolution of which is little known—escape treatment and follow-up, probably due to the self-healing tendency of this form.

The Localized Polar Paucibacillary Form

> The paradox of the polar paucibacillary (PP) or TT form of Hansen's disease, while indicating a hyperergic state of the host with high levels of specific cell-mediated immunity that ultimately destroys and clears the invading organism in the tissues, concomitant nerve damage is often the case as a result of delayed hypersensitivity (DHR) to antigenic components.[20]

True PP (TT) form of Hansen's disease is quite rare, in that a reported 75% of this form of the disease undergoes spontaneous recovery in the absence of chemotherapy and within some five years of detection, and as such shows no particular interest, as has been pointed out.

As the classical high immune and stable end of the disease spectrum, PP (TT) form of the disease implies—apart from zero bacillary load and positive late Mitsuda reaction—resistance or cell-mediated immunity indicated by a granulomatous inflammation or immunological granuloma,[21] the clinical evidence of which is shown by the limitation of disease and appearance of well-defined margins plus healing center among skin lesions, as indicated by Bryceson (1981).

The hallmark of PP (TT) form of Hansen's disease is the immunological granuloma and, to a variable extent, equally of the borderline paucibacillary (BP) or BT and borderline (BB) forms of the disease. As the focal, non-specific expression of the immune response, the immunological granuloma indicates that, in PP (TT) form, the host has acquired a vigorous cell-mediated immunity (CMI) and, besides, developed delayed hypersensitivity (DHR) to Hansen's bacillus (*M. leprae*) and its antigens, though at a price. Such a granulomatous inflammation bears on the granuloma per se and the cellular infiltrate:

- The main characteristics of the immunological granuloma (viz. cell type, bacterial load, nerve and skin involvement) suggest that they are consequent to delayed hypersensitivity (DHR) to Hansen's bacillus (*M. leprae*) and its antigens.

  Histology shows highly differentiated, blood-borne, tightly-packed granuloma cells—or lumped macrophages[22]—epithelioid cells[23] and, perhaps, Langhans' giant cells.

  The pathogenesis of the focal, non-specific expression of the immune response or immunological granuloma is best illustrated by the diagram below in keeping with the views of Ridley (1985): As regards Hansen's disease, the immunological granuloma always signifies either the site of the bacillus or the site of its destruction (Ridley and Job, 1985). Apart from indicating that the host has acquired a vigorous resistance and developed delayed hypersensitivity (DHR) to the bacillus and its antigens, the immunological granuloma is a response whereby prevention of further cellular multiplication and spread of the organism is the case (Lagrange and Hurtrel, 1986). Moreover, the immunological granuloma develops only after recognition of antigen (Ridley and

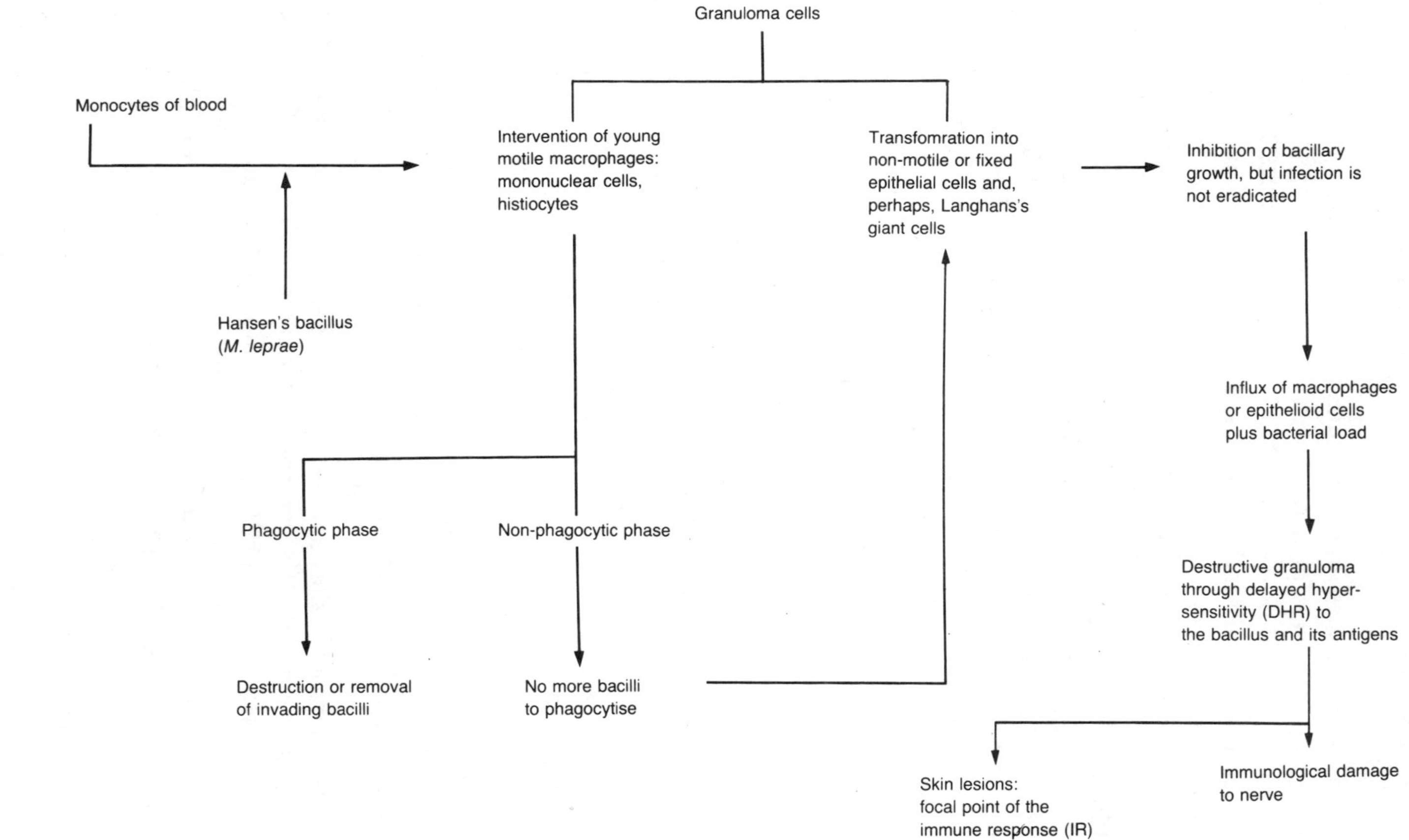

Monocytes of blood
Hansen's bacillus
(M. leprae)
Granuloma cells
Intervention of young motile macrophages: mononuclear cells, histiocytes
Transfomration into non-motile or fixed epithelial cells and, perhaps, Langhans's giant cells
Inhibition of bacillary growth, but infection is not eradicated
Influx of macrophages or epithelioid cells plus bacterial load
Destructive granuloma through delayed hyper-sensitivity (DHR) to the bacillus and its antigens
Phagocytic phase
Non-phagocytic phase
Destruction or removal of invading bacilli
No more bacilli to phagocytise
Skin lesions: focal point of the immune response (IR)
Immunological damage to nerve

Job, 1985), and is at the onset a non-specific feature that is frequently undistinguishable from the one relating to, for instance, granuloma multiforme, lupus vulgaris, or sarcoidosis, notwithstanding schistosomiasis, cutaneous leishmaniasis, and tuberculosis, mentioned equally by Goihman-Yar (1980).

The immunological granuloma, as has been intimated, is localized by way of selective involvement of the so-called protected sites more or less peculiar to Hansen's disease, these, in order of importance, being: nerve bundles, erector pili muscle, epidermis or sub-epidermal zone, sweat glands,[24] and neurovascular bundles. Any one of those protected sites is besides, liable to be involved by the bacillus, immunological granuloma, or cellular infiltrate in that order of importance.

Common to both nerve and skin involvement, the immunological granuloma is highly organized and makes its first appearance in deep nerve bundles of the sub-epidermal zone (cf. sub-papillary plexus of vessels in the superficial dermis), through which spread and dissemination take place (Ridley, 1985). From that zone, the immunological granuloma extends to the neurovascular bundle of the sub-epidermis, or infiltration occurs between the collagen bundles of the dermis (Ridley, 1985). When fully established and increased in size, the immunological granuloma can fill almost the entire dermis at one site through infiltration or expansion, or both, as stated by the author.

Nerve involvement by the immunological granuloma is more important than involvement of epidermis or sweat glands, the finding of Hansen's bacillus (*M. leprae*), in clumps or parallel to the axons, being diagnostic of the disease. Disorientation of Schwann cells and disorganization of nerve structure or perineurium is strong evidence of the disease, and presence of the bacillus or immunological granuloma, diagnostic (Fleury and Bacchi, 1987).

Two events in the peripheral nerve are noteworthy: (i) sooner or later, in the absence of early diagnostic and/or chemotherapy, the formation of a destructive immunological granuloma with its expected sequelae; (ii) the probable invasion of the whole endoneurial zone by granuloma cells at the periphery of the nerve bundle, followed by the breaching of the perineurial barrier as a result of colonization of perineurial cells by Hansen's bacillus (*M.*

leprae), as intimated by Ridley (1985). This being the case, adds the author, bacilli break out beyond it in the dermis where they establish themselves.

- Upon regression, the epithelioid cells of the immunological granuloma die and macrophage undergo morphological changes, the overall result, following chemotherapy, being a non-specific cellular infiltrate known to obscure diagnosis and classification of the disease as has been mentioned by Ridley (1985).

The cellular infiltrate, the other component of the inflammatory reaction, precedes the appearance of the immunological granuloma in the lesion and persists, as stated above, as the result of regression. The infiltrate consist mostly of small round cells or lymphocytes, or turf of surrounding lymphocytes,[25] and histiocytes or fibrocytes, none of them, incidentally, host cells to Hansen's bacillus (*M. leprae*), quite a relevant point.

The cellular infiltrate, while surrounding or encapsulating the nests or foci made up by granuloma cells, is diagnostically less reliable than the immunological granuloma as recalled by Ridley (1985). Lymphocytes are reportedly quite numerous in the immunological granuloma, their distribution comprising T-helper cells predominantly (i.e., diffusely distributed among aggregated epithelioid cells and the periphery), most of these expressing the OKT 4 + subset or surface phenotype of helper (The) cells, and a few suppressor (Ts) cells confined mainly to the periphery of the lesion, together with corresponding OKT 8 + subset or surface phenotype of suppressor (Ts) and cytotoxic cells.[26]

In their study of the immunological granuloma in Hansen's disease, Rea and Modlin (1987) found that helper T-cells were four times as numerous in PP (TT) lesions as in PM (LL) lesions.[27]

Furthermore, there is a decrease of helper T-cells and a reduction of the ratio helper/suppressor T lymphocytes from PP (TT) to the PM (LL) spectrum of the disease as demonstrated by van Voorhis et al. (1982) and, subsequently, by other authors.[28]

The immune-mediated tissue involvement in paucibacillary (PP) or TT form of Hansen's disease implies:

This is an early feature confined to only one or a few peripheral nerves in the presence of the immunological granuloma as the source of nerve damage mild to moderate in nature.[29] However, nerve damage is preceded by neuritis, two features that are incidentally not synonymous, in that, as pointed out by Job (1989), there can be neuritis with little or no evidence of nerve damage, and nerve damage can occur through some other causes.

Neuritis or inflammation of the peripheral nerve is always found in all forms of Hansen's disease, admittedly in a unique way, the end-stage of which being perineurial fibrosis and hyalinization of the nerve parenchyma leading to the destruction of nerves on, unfortunately, a permanent, irreversible basis.

The ensuing neuritis of only one or a few peripheral (motor) nerve trunks is characterized by swelling, edema, and compression of those nerves within the endoneurium, hence leading to motor weakness and wasting of muscle. If the sheath is unyielding, the pathological process involves considerable destruction with associated enlargement of the nerve trunks, motor paralysis present or not. Depending on the type of nerve involved, caseation may give rise to a sterile nerve abscess. Bacilli, whenever present, are almost invariably found in the Schwann cells.

As regards the sensory and autonomic[30] nerves, their terminal twigs are obliterated within and around the perineurium. Nerves within the infiltrate are either destroyed or greatly swollen, as has been pointed out. About 30% of sensory fibres must reportedly be destroyed before there is any evidence of sensory impairment, which, in this case, is usually marked (viz. insensitivity, sensory loss, or anesthesia) and more often than not accompanied by anhydrosis (lack of sweating), deficiency of hair growth in the affected areas, and enlargement of cutaneous nerves in the vicinity of skin lesions.

Whilst, from a clinical viewpoint, muscle atrophy and/or paralysis begs the obvious by virtue of its sheer visual impact, let it be recalled that insensitivity of the skin or sensory loss is the most insidious and foremost complication of Hansen's disease, the main predisposing factor of secondary infection, the major mediator of disability and/or deformity as has been previously discussed.

Of particular interest at this stage is the pure neural form of

Hansen's disease or primary polyneuritis whereby the infection is localized to the primary intraneural focus, as remarked by Stoner (1981).

Primary polyneuritis is not solely confined to other endemic countries other than Africa, as believed in some quarters, the present writer vouching for the contrary. Of late, Berhan (1989) reported a total of 83 patients showing, admittedly, that unusual presentation in Ethiopia, i.e, a clinical entity without any skin lesions, its histological features consistent with PP (TT) form of Hansen's disease and borderline paucibacillary (BP) or BT.[31]

The reason put forward why the skin is spared is that, being a primary, self-contained infection within Schwann cells, no surviving bacilli or their antigens can escape from the nerve into the neighboring skin to trigger, in turn, a cellular reaction. Although spontaneous regression may occur earlier on in primary polyneuritis, in either case the ulnar nerve is the most commonly affected, asymmetrically so, alone or at times in association with other peripheral nerves. Clinically, the nerve(s) may be tender and uniformly enlarged, with or without abscess formation brought about by caseation. Sensory changes are often marked more than motor changes, touch and temperature being the first to be affected, pressure and pain next.

As result, early manifestations of the neuropathy are paresthesia, numbness, muscle weakness, and neuralgia following acute inflammation of the nerve. Late manifestations include paresis, hypotonia, atrophy of the muscle of hand and foot, and eventually—if not checked in time—claw hand and wrist drop, and claw toes and foot drop with attendant trophic changes.

Skin lesions

As Jopling (1984) pointed out, once the surviving bacilli or their antigens escape from Schwann cells into adjoining skin (details of which were taken up subsequently by Ridley), a cellular reaction takes place, i.e., a skin lesion is likely to develop at that site from a perivascular immunological granuloma. In fact, as already intimated, the first step in the inception of a skin lesion is via the presence of Hansen's bacillus (*M. leprae*) in Schwann cells, its habitat. Outside that protected site, though, there is no barrier to antigen recognition and the immunological granuloma forms without delay over the entire area of recognition, as expressed by Ridley et al. (1986), consisting, as is the case with the peripheral nerve, of both immunological granuloma and cellular infiltrate around, this time, skin appendages or adnexa,[32] with or without invasion of the sub-papillary zone, with or without erosion of the basal layer of the dermis.

Skin lesions are the morphological expression of the immune response, in that for many immunologists, notably Godal (1984), there is considerable evidence suggesting that the immune response to Hansen's bacillus (*M. leprae*) is the major cause of those lesions, including other tissues. For other authors, should the skin be the portal of entry of the bacillus—particularly in the PP (LL) form of the disease—and established beyond doubt, then it would be reasonable to assume that the cutaneous infiltrates of the hansenians (leprosy patients) are indeed the primary site of the host immune response to Hansen's bacillus (*M. leprae*).

Skin lesions or cutaneous infiltrate in PP (TT) form of the disease[33] are clinically macular and plague-like, often single or few in number, asymmetrical and with well-defined and unbroken margin as a rule, a healing center often the case. As previously stated, owing to involvement of sensory and autonomic nerve fibres, the surface of these lesions is insensitive, hairless, and dry.

Skin lesions on the face are, incidentally, much less insensitive than those elsewhere, on account of the rich overlapping of nerve supply to that area, as has been remarked.

Immunologically-Mediated Complications or Reactions

By contrast to borderline paucibacillary (BP) or BT and PM (LL) forms of Hansen's disease, immunologically-mediated complications or reactional states are not the features as a rule of PP (TT) form, depending, though, on whether there is any antigen left to be uncovered in the view of Ridley (1985).

The Disseminated Polar Multibacillary Form

> Basically an immunodeficiency disease or anergic state,[34] polar multibacillary (PM) or LL form of Hansen's disease is, apart from its infectivity, the chief concern at all levels.

The majority of patients belonging to the PM (LL) form of the disease[35] have downgraded from the borderline or interpolar group—actually, mostly BB and BL—thus indicating a declining resistance to infection brought about further on by the inability of the host to mount a cell-mediated immunity to Hansen's bacillus (*M. leprae*) and its antigens. Possible explanations for it having already been discussed, suffice it to say that such a failure or deficiency is made manifest by the spread of the disease process, absence of immunological granuloma, helper T-cell depletion, and a negative Mitsuda reaction.

As stated by Jopling (1984), those bacilli, liberated or released extra-cellularly when Schwann cells and perineurial cells are destroyed, are engulfed by histiocytes (macrophages) which, instead of destroying them and becoming fixed or non-mobile epithelioid cells as in the case with PP (TT) form of the disease, become wandering macrophages allowing Hansen's bacillus (*M. leprae*) to multiply within them, hence reaching skin and other tissues or organs via the blood stream (systemic route).

Macrophages, in the words of Ridley (1983), being "the ideal host to the bacillus they should have destroyed, (remaining) the most important constituents of every lepromatous lesion," it follows that, in contrast to the PP (TT) form of the disease, the focal point here is the non-immunological or macrophage granuloma or "leproma" usually described as a diffuse cellular response consisting of foamy, poorly differentiated, or undifferentiated macrophages on account of the fatty changes undergone by their cytoplasm in the shape of large vacuolated histiocytes or Virchow's cells, also known as "lepra cells," bacilli isolated or in globi with a few of them surrounding lymphocytes or none. In other words, the non-immunological macrophage granuloma comprises sheets of macrophages loaded with bacilli along with plasma cells and a few lymphocytes diffusely distributed into the granuloma, as described by Ridley (1985).

The author, moreover, points out that in the non-immunological macrophage granuloma, the more the multiplication of bacilli, the greater the influx of healthy young macrophages. Yet, upon slowing down the multiplication of those bacilli and consequently the influx of young macrophages with, concurrently, death and degeneration of many organisms, the fat content of the cytoplasm continues to increase, the soapy appearance is more marked, small vesicles develop and coalesce to form vacuoles. The larger the vacuole the higher the proportion of fat, and the lower the proportion of bacilli within: a macrophage granuloma where the majority of macrophages are marked fatty changes is a sign of regression, the latter hastened by chemotherapy.

Nerve involvement implies bacillation of the vascular endoneurial cells by Hansen's bacillus (*M. leprae*), even the perineurium being no longer acting as an immunological barrier and whose "onion peel" appearance in the dermal nerve is due to infiltration by histiocytes and plasma cells, as intimated by Bryceson and Pfaltzgraff (1979).

In the skin, the histological picture reveals a thin epidermis, flattened rete ridges, and a clear zone in which bacilli are rarely found (Jopling, 1984). Or, as Ridley and Job (1985) put it with fuller details:

- macrophage granuloma with no epithelioid cells and not very many small lymphocytes, foamy changes in variable amount;
- small or large vacuoles in the cytoplasm when regression sets in;
- nerve fairly normal or with onion-skin perineurium but with significant infiltration, or fairly normal;
  AFB = 5 − 6 +

The antigens expressed on the lymphocyte membranes are, in this case, OKT 8 + (subset or surface genotype or suppressor (Ts) cells and cytotoxic cells) found in the non-immunological granuloma, though, according to Harboe (1985), there is no separation of OKT 4 + and OKT 8 + in that they are distributed throughout the granuloma.

In the view of van Voorhis, et al. (1982), the presence of the above subsets of surface phenotypes may suppress the alleged function of OKT 4 + cells (i.e., their stimulation of T-cells lympholines), or may act directly to suppress macrophage activation.

Although nerves are not the sites of high bacillary concentration as is the skin, here the type of nerve damage, secondary to perineurial damage, is unique in Hansen's disease, different from the immuno-pathological process in other forms of the disease, much slower to manifest itself as well known.

In contrast to PP (TT) form of the disease, nerve involvement in PM (LL) form is symmetrical on the whole, with at first surprisingly little damage to the nerve fiber despite the bacillary load. Terminal nerve twigs are damaged more easily than nerve trunks through a very gradual process of hyaline degeneration and fibrosis over several years as generally acknowledged.

The overall picture is that of a slow-going peripheral neuropathy, involvement of numerous peripheral nerves following an impressive bacillary infiltration, with nerve damage a symmetrical phenomenon, one side, though, liable to be affected earlier than the other, as has been remarked.

Clinically, one sees an initial enlargement and tenderness, ultimately bilateral thinness and hardness due to edema and constrictive fibrosis or compression neuropathy depending on which nerves are involved. The end result is sensory and motor deficit with their attendant sequelae: anhydrosis of the affected skin, excessive sweating of the non-affected areas, "glove-and-stocking" anesthesia in advanced cases, shortening of digits due to painless and repeated trauma, gross facial deformities or leonine facies, and ocular pathology up to blindness.

Skin Lesions

Skin lesions dominated by the non-immunological macrophage granuloma are strikingly symmetrical, not anesthetic initially, and it is—as Jopling (1984) observed—through gradual extension of nerve damage over the years that total anesthesia of the limbs and trunk finally occurs. The early skin lesions are widely distributed: very numerous macules, non-anesthetic at first, erythematous on light skin and coppery on dark skin as Jopling (1984) stated, ill-defined margins and shiny surface. Papules and nodules showing a great variety of sizes and color follow.

Thickening and nodulation of both ears are early manifestations which, allowed to progress untreated, lead to generalized infiltration and thickness of the affected parts,[37] especially the cheeks, forehead, and ear lobes, giving rise—as mentioned above—to the classical leonine facies with nodular masses and collapse of the bridge of the nose, hoarseness of the voice, and loss of the upper incisors. Both superciliary and ciliary madarosis, chronic edema of legs[38] during the day, and accompanying tenderness on palpation are frequently the case.[39]

Other Tissues and Organs

In many PM (LL) patients, invasion of the nasal mucosa of the nose with resulting nasal stuffiness, crust formation, and epistaxis may be among the first symptoms, as pointed out by Jopling (1984).

Eye, bone, and testicular pathological involvement as a systemic phenomenon contribute to the complications of that form of the disease and imply that many deep tissues and organs are invaded by bacillated macrophages, too. Severe tissue damage is due to a confrontation between antibody and antigen with the production of circulatory immune complexes[40] leading to cutaneous ulcerations, uveitis, and glomerulo-nephritis as has been written about.

Immunologically-Mediated Complications or Reactions

The immunologically-mediated complications or reactional states occurring in PP (LL) form of the disease[41] follow the same basic principle as the one that will be met in the borderline group: an allergic inflammatory process not an essential part of the infective process of Hansen's disease, through it may often be associated with either its spread or resolution (Ridley, 1985).

The subject, as very well known by now, bears on three complications or reactions: (i) erythema nodosum hansenicum (leprosum) or ENH (ENL) (Jopling's Type II); (ii) Lucio phenomenon, the mediators in both of these being circulating immune complexes;[42] and (iii) exacerbation reactions[43]:

- As a classical example of immune complex disease,[44] erythema nodosum hansenicum (leprosum) or ENH (ENL) usually occurs during the phase of regression following treatment, though reportedly rarely so except, for instance, in Brazil, where many hansenians report to their physicians on account of their ENL in the absence of initial therapy.[45] From Ridley (1985):

The induction of this immunologically-mediated reaction depends on the nature of the antigen-antibody ration, the latter probably an important determinant of the size of the lesions and antigen deposit engaged in reaction. Although an acknowledged entity, erythema nodosum hansenicum (leprosum) or ENH (ENL), shows more apparent histological than clinical variants with marked ethnic bias.

(i) Thus in the classical form of ENH (ENL), the pink type, the reaction is centered on a small old regressing non-immunological macrophage granuloma in the sub-epidermis with a polymorph infiltration, i.e., a cluster of polymorph neutrophils around accumulation of foamy cells. Vasculitis is not a conspicuous feature or, if present, a secondary one. Scanty or degenerated AFB, bacterial debris, and components for immune complex formation[46] are demonstrable at the site, both extracellularly and in polymorphs.

(ii) The more severe reaction, necrotizing ENH (ENL),[47] is similar but involves a larger regressive granulomatous site with probably more AFB on display, a more severe vasculitis.

(iii) Other than the polymorph infiltration of the granuloma, involvement of dermal connective tissue is occasionally more conspicuous.[48] When mild in nature, it is characterized by edema of the dermal connective tissue; when severe, it consists of fibrinoid necrosis, elastosis, and infiltration of fibroblasts followed by intensive fibrosis. Blood vessels may also be involved by way of severe subacute vasculitis in the absence of haemorrahage or thrombosis. As expressed by Ridley next:

- Lucio phenomenon,[49] a reaction considered as an acute allergic vasculitis, its pathogenesis less well understood yet confined almost exclusively to Mexico and Central America, is actually a diffuse PM (LL) form of Hansen's disease characterized by capillary endothelium of the sub-papillary plexus by AFB, which, upon breaking down, leads to hemorrhage and epidermal infarction. Deeper in the dermis, large granulomatous masses show an acute inflammation similar to ENH (ENL). Components of the immune complex are demonstrated in the wall of the blood vessels and in the perivascular areas. Finally:

- Distinct from erythema nodosum hansenicum (leprosum) or ENH (ENL) and other forms of reactions, localized without systemic effects at the sites of the largest and most active lesions, and not immunologically-mediated complications, exacerbation reactions are characterized by a polymorph infiltrate probably associated with macrophage degeneration and, more importantly, an exceptional bacterial load. In advanced cases, severe edema, exudation, local hemorrhage, and necrosis of small capillaries in the central area occur as signs of increased capillary permeability.

Clinically, as advocated by Pfaltzgraff (1989), it is preferable to use the term erythema nodosum hansenicum (leprosum) or ENL (ENH) when solely as a humoral response in the skin; the term Type 2 reserved for any humoral reaction involving nerves, joints, eyes, etc., including ENH (ENL).

The Fluctuating Interpolar Group

By virtue of its shifting immunological status, the interpolar or borderline group of Hansen's disease occupies a large central portion of the disease spectrum, and as such its highly complex nature implies an evolutionary stage of the two polar forms of the disease.

As a result of changes in their immunological status or shifting cell-mediated immunity (CMI), the interpolar or borderline group of Hansen's disease is aptly described by Bryceson (1981) as symbolizing "battles between the protective effects of cell-mediated immunity and the immuno-suppressive effects of antigenic load." The immunological instability of the group by reason of a shifting CMI means an upgrading reaction in the case of borderline paucibillary (BP) or BT, and the downgrading in respect of borderline multibacillary (BM) or BL.

One is reminded by Bryceson (1981) that most patients at diagnosis are either BP (BT) or BM (BL) and "the instability which allows them to move within the spectrum, is probably determined by the effects of the bacillary load upon the immune response." In short, as has been pointed out, a disturbance of the pre-existing immunological balance that brings about a bewildering array of clinical manifestations.

- Borderline borderline (BB) as such is quite rare on account of its notorious instability, i.e., as the center of the disease spectrum it hinges—as has been remarked—on a delicate and precarious balance between bacillary multiplication and cellular immunity.

The important characteristic of this form is the tendency to reactional episode, which is accompanied by rapid changes to nerve and skin through an acute cellular hypersensitivity, as has been pointed out.

According to Ridley and Job (1985), the immunological granuloma is present with "fairly scanty and diffuse lymphocytes, and no Langhans's giant cells. Nerves are greatly swollen and may be normal or lamination of the perineurium with invading epithelioid cells may be present. The subepidermal zone is clear, edema is a common feature here," besides moderate AFB, negative smears and Mitsuda reaction.

Peripheral neuropathy is moderate, though many nerves can be affected in an asymmetrical pattern. On the other hand, the condition may be a purely neuritic one in early stages. Enlargement of the nerve may be regular, or not. Sensory loss or insensitivity is equally moderate, yet an equally early phenomenon, too, as has been altogether reported.

Dermal lesions are few or numerous with a tendency to symmetry, well-defined or poorly so. Satellite lesions are common, and other lesions annular with a punched-out appearance, i.e., vague border and a clearly marked inner border, as is well known.

- Borderline paucibacillary (BP) or BT represents the peak of acute nerve damage in Hansen's disease through a pre-existing intense cellular infiltrate, the extent of which is a predisposing factor of much importance, as has been intimated elsewhere.

As described by Ridley and Job (1985), the immunological granuloma shows "a moderate number of lympocytes, or small nondescript Langhans's giant cells. The nerve is swollen with lymphocytes with slight lamination, or occasionally no more than a spike of infiltration or erosion of the dermis, or variable infiltration of the sub-epidermal zone." AFB: 0-2 +.

Peripheral neuropathy is more common here, and more frequent than in the PP (TT) form of the disease, i.e., widespread and asymmetrical, numerous peripheral nerve trunks irregularly enlarged, almost all of them in longstanding cases, with corresponding sensory loss or paresis often at the outset. As indicated earlier on, BP (BT) patients may turn up as primary polyneuritic form in the absence of cutaneous lesions.

Clinically, involvement of peripheral nerves in order of frequency means: ulnar, median, facial, lateral popliteal or common peroneal, posterior tibial, and radial nerves.

Skin lesions imply macules or plaques not so large as in PP (TT), but more numerous, insensitive, asymmetrical, with a less dry surface and less clear-cut margins. Hair growth is less affected, and satellite lesions may be present. Skin smears are usually negative and the Mitsuda reaction weakly positive.

- As one would expect, the features of borderline multibacillary (BM) or BL are attributable in a mixed way to bacillary invasion and instability, these two together being responsible for the rapid downhill progress of this sub-type towards the PM (LL) form of the disease with its attendant complications, as has been put forward.

This explains why an overwhelming proportion of PM or BL patients shown some evidence of the earlier borderline phase, as has been reported. Once more, Ridley and Job (1985) tell us that the non-immunological macrophage granuloma presents with numerous lymphocytes densely packed over the whole of at least one segment with or without lymphocytes, or a combination of moderate numbers of lymphocytes and undifferentiated granuloma cells. There are some foamy changes, but no vacuoles in the macrophages. Nerves commonly show an onion-skin perineurium. AFB: 4-5 +, and Mitsuda reaction negative.

Peripheral neuropathy is characterized by enlarged nerves in a widespread and symmetrical way upon appearance of skin lesions, but with slight sensory loss and muscle weakness, i.e., little nerve dysfunction, and unlikelihood of nerve damage as rapid as in BB and BP or BT.

Skin lesions are numerous, not distributed absolutely symmetrically, differing in size and shape. Macules, papules, plaques, and nodules may all be present, yet not so shiny and succulent. Other features like madarosis, keratitis, nasal ulceration, etc., so typical of PM or BL are absent, as has been described.

The main immunologically-mediated complications or reactions that occur mostly in the BP (BT)–BM (BL) range of Hansen's disease spectrum,[50] or "reversal" (cf. Jopling's Type 1) reaction due to activation of cell-mediated immunity, are almost certainly the result of a flare-up of delayed hypersensitivity (DHR) to Hansen's bacillus (*M. leprae*) and its antigens, i.e., a reaction associated with cell-mediated hypersensitivity and leaving an innocent victim: immune-mediated tissue involvement meaning loss of nerve function and, if unchecked, deformities peculiar to the disease.

While, in the view of Mshana and Nilsen (1988), it in not clear what triggers that sudden flare-up of delayed hypersensitivity (DHR) and whether it is directed at the specific antigens of the bacillus or not, such an episode is the primary cause of morbidity of the disease.

By contrast, the opinion of Ridley (1985) is that DHR seems to be triggered off either by a rise in the level of hypersensitivity or an increase in the load of immunologically detected antigens at a particular site or sites. Alternately, instead of an increase, there may be an uncovering of previously undetected antigen—in a nerve, for example—which may itself come about as a result of increased hypersensitivity.[51]

Of late, the study of intralesional and cellular immunoregulatory events in "reversal" or Jopling's Type 1 reaction by Scollard et al. (1989) indicates, in the view of the authors, that "the likely mechanism (for that reaction) involves transient or intermittent activation of T-helper cells, together with their recruitment and proliferation with the lesion."

Prior to clinical appearance of DHR, the histological picture reveals the possibility of (i) some diffuse extracellular in and around the immunological granuloma and in the superficial dermis and (ii) a diffuse proliferation of fibrocytes in the dermis which, in this case, is unrelated to the granuloma itself. In the early stage of DHR, a cellular influx associated with it causes an infiltrative spread in addition. When clinically evident, the picture varies greatly in degree, edema and proliferation of fibrocytes being possibly profuse or barely significant, with or without the presence of foreign body vacuolated[52] as described by Ridley (1985).

The author pursues that, whereas in the acute reactional phase a breakdown and dispersal of the immunological granuloma takes place, even liquefaction necrosis and ulceration (i) terminates with the development of PM (LL) granuloma if the reaction proves downgrading in the first place.

Notes

1. By Gerhard Armauer Hansen in the 1870s, i.e., some sixty years before a suitable animal model was found for research purposes and some seventy years before the appearance of the first suitable treatment of the disease, as remarked by Kaufmann et al. (1986).
2. Whereas Shepard worked out the density of bacilli per gram of tissue (viz. a fantastic 10^{10}), the non-toxicity of the organism is explained by the fact that as a result, there are no side effects. This also explains, according to Harboe (1985), its capacity to hinder recognition but trigger immuno-suppression.
3. I.e., resists cultivation on artificial media. As Dhople (1988) puts it: "Cultivation of the responsible microorganism is almost a prerequisite for the control of most infectious diseases. The cultivation of *M. leprae* remains one of the last frontiers in this area of microbiology and has provided both a challenge as well as a feeling of despair. Unfortunately, not many laboratories are involved in cultivation work. The number of scientists working in this area is diminishing year by year. What is the reason? Are the younger scientists frightened of the diseases or do they feel that their careers will be threatened if they don't get fast results or are we discouraging them with the controversies which have surrounded previous claims of cultivation of *M. leprae*? It is high time that responsible persons and agencies look into this matter seriously."
4. I.e., the capacity of Hansen's bacillus (*M. leprae*), when strained with carbol fuchsin (red dye), to retain its red color upon treatment with acid. However, as pointed out by Rees (1985), the acid fastness of the majority of bacilli, though strong in nature, is irregular; only in the minority of the organisms is it uniform.
5. Hence indicating the predominant role of the host in determining the type of the disease (Rotberg, 1937; Rees,1985).
6. With a molecular basis related to the cell wall composition, actually a peptide glycogen to which are attached polysaccharide chains bearing mycotic acids,

these thought to be associated with the stimulation of delayed hypersensitivity (DHR).

7. Cf. a generation time of 12 to 14 days during its logarithmic phase of growth, followed by a dormant phase where it remains viable for years without going into cell division as stated by Haregewoin (1985).

8. In the view of Kato (1968).

9. Hansen's bacillus (*M. leprae*) has a substantial number of antigenic molecules, a majority of which cross-react with other mycobacteria, and PM (LL) patients produce antibodies to most of these molecules, as indicated by Mshana and Nilsen (1988).

10. Newell (1966) quotes Hamilton (1929) (cuts); Knolkar (1955) (intact skin); Dowell (1967) (wounds). Rotberg (1988), following a personal communication to the present writer, quotes Porrit and Olsen (1947) (tattooed U.S. Marines). This view is accepted nowadays by Ridley and Job (1985), Bryceson (1985), Machin (1988), and Job (1988).

11. Quoted by Hastings (1988).

12. Jopling (1984), Noordeen (1985), Languillon (1986), McDougall and Yamalkar (1987), Waters (1988).

13. I.e., the axis cylinder conducting impulses.

14. Eleven to eighteen days in the foot-pads of normal mice versus twenty minutes for *M. tuberculosis* (Rees, 1985).

15. The Ridley-Jopling scale has the great advantage of grouping the various types (polar) and sub-types (interpolar or borderline) of Hansen's disease according to their immune status as judged by clinical criteria, histological evidence and bacteriology, and response to the Mitsuda ("lepromin") reaction. A whole spectrum, in other words, having an important bearing on the conduct of chemotherapy, prognosis of the disease, and the usefulness of such a scale in research trials as altogether expounded by Ridley (1985).

16. The indeterminate (Idt) was proposed at the International Leprosy Congress in Havanna, 1948, and sanctioned at the following Congress in Madrid, 1953.

17. Pettit (1981) queries whether Idt should ever be diagnosed, hence his plea that the term be banished from scientific vocabulary and, in reply, the considered opinion of Browne (1982) to the contrary.

18. The inception or initial involvement of Hansen's disease is via the Schwann cells, the target organ of the bacillus.

19. I.e., the non-vascular elements or nerve fibers in the plexus of the dermis.

20. Or Type IV in the Gell and Coombs' classification of immunologically-mediated mechanisms of tissue damage.

21. The term granuloma was first introduced by Virchow as a tumor mass or nodule of granulation and defined by Turk as a localized collection of cells of the mononuclear phagocyte system with or without the admixture of other inflammatory cell types (quoted by Narayanan et al., 1988). The designation "immunological" granuloma used by Ridley et al. (1986) is adopted here.

22. Let it be recalled that macrophages are involved in antigen presentation and elicitation of the immune response. As regards granuloma cells, they are tumor-like cells and have, as would be expected, different life spans: the shortest in respect of Langhans's giant cells, the longest in favor of macrophages in active and non-active lesions, epithelioid cells in between, as described by Ridley (1985).

23. Typical mononuclear phagocytes and part of the reticulo-endothelial system, the

exact function of which is not known. The relationship between epithelioid cells and macrophages was recognized by Metchikoff in the early 1880s as reported by Narayanan et al. (1988).

24. For reasons unknown, infiltration and destruction of sweat glands are not a feature of PM (LL) form of the disease, as pointed out by Ridley and Job (1985).

25. The maximal density of which is being found in PP (TT) form of the disease, followed by downgrading in the interpolar or borderline group, and minimally so in PM (LL) form.

26. T-cell population is divided into functionally distinct groups according to the molecules they exhibit on their surface membranes. The two most notable antigens expressed on the lympocytes' membrane being OKT 4 + (helper T-cell), comprising about 65% of all T lymphocytes, the remaining 35% being OKT 8 + (suppressor cells and cytotoxic cells). These predominant T-cell sub-sets or surface phenotypes suggest that they may be specialized to activate lymphokines' production, these, in turn, stimulating macrophage activation and hence limiting bacillary growth and the extent of dermal involvement, as intimated by Ridley and Job (1985).

27. Quoted by Hastings (1987).

28. Ridley, Russell, and Ridley (1982); Modlin et al. (1983); Narayanan et al. (1983); Longley et al. (1985) quoted by Flad et al. (1988).

29. Described by Fleury and Bacchi (1987) as (i) dense infiltration of inflammatory cells in the endoneurium and (ii) endoneurium granuloma of nerve branches inside the granuloma, thus permitting (iii) the identification of PP (TT) form of the disease over other types of non-specific granulomas.

30. Nerve controlling, inter alia, blood vessels independently of the will, as recalled by Jopling (1984).

31. Also observed in the interpolar or borderline patients by Cochrane and Khanolkar, as quoted by Ridley and Job (1985).

32. Viz. the pilo-sebaceous units plus eccrine and apocrine glands endowed with a rich network of nerves and blood vessels.

33. For a more detailed and authoritative description of skin lesions in Hansen's disease, vide: *Leprosy*, edited by R. C. Hastings (Churchill Livingstone, 1985) and Languillon's *Précis de Léprologie* (2nd Edition, Masson, Paris, 1986).

34. First described by von Pirquet, in 1911, as the antipode of allergy, a probably determined genetical state. It implies, by now, rather a failure to form a mature immunological granuloma in response to the antigens of Hansen's bacillus (*M. leprae*), or a disturbance in the dynamic equilibrium between helper (Th) T-cells and suppressor (Ts) T-cells activity seen in both cell-mediated immunity and DHR, as remarked by Maier (1987).

35. Little is known about the nature of antibodies that occur in this form of the disease, particularly to which structural components of the bacillus they are directed against (Goihman-Yar, 1980). It seems that PM (LL) form is associated with high levels of relevant and irrelevant antibodies as well as autoantibodies (Maier, 1987).

36. Ridley (1983).

37. Through aggregation of granulomatous tissue.

38. The invasion of capillaries (endothelial walls) by Hansen's bacillus (*M. leprae*), combined with damage to dermal nerves controlling those capillaries, causes increased capillary permeability, which, combined in turn with the effect of gravity, results in edema (Jopling, 1984).

39. Incidentally, alopecia is not, as pointed out by Jopling (1984), a proven feature of Hansen's disease, but ichthyosis (thighs, legs, arm, or trunk) may be a late manifestation.

40. Cf. polymorphic nuclear infiltration, endarteritis, hyaline degeneration of media of small arterioles, and intra-arterial thrombosis.

41. Whereas quite well documented elsewhere (cf. Bryceson and Pfaltzgraff, 1979 and 1981; Jopling, 1984; Languillon, 1986; Pfaltzgraff and Bryceson, 1985). Ridley (1985) reminds us that such complications or reactions are somewhat confused both in concept and nomenclature, on account of the underlying allergic inflammatory process which, not an essential part of the infective process of Hansen's disease—even though it may be associated with either its spread or resolution—present in much the same way clinically regardless of its cause, hence the ensuing difficulty in elucidating the reaction on clinical grounds, or even differentiating it from relapse.

    Of late, Pfaltzgraff (1989) is of the opinion that there is still a good deal of confusion about the subject of reactions in Hansen's disease, in that, although immunologically determined, their basic mechanism(s) is not fully understood. For convenience's sake, pursues the author, Type I reaction of the interpolar or borderline group is the cellular response of the individual to antigens of the bacillus, while corresponding to Type IV in the Gell and Coombs' classification of immunologically-mediated mechanisms of tissue damage. Type 2 reaction of PM (LL) form of the disease is the humoral response of the individual to antigens of the bacillus, while corresponding to Gell and Coombs' type III (immune complex).

42. As Harboe (1985) states, release of mycobacterial antigens from the macrophages is required for the formation of circulating immune complexes.

43. Histologically similar but immunologically distinct.

44. The immunological findings and the data supporting such a concept are somehow weaker by now than previously thought in the view of Harboe (1985), in that the pathogenesis of ENH (ENL) may be more complex and other immunological mechanisms may be involved as well. The condition is, incidentally, found in tuberculosis, sarcoidosis, post-streptococcal infection, deep fungal infection, inflammatory bowel disease, Yersinia enterocolitis, pregnancy; it can also be idiopathic, or drug-related.

45. Personal communication from Rotberg (1988).

46. Mycobacterial antigen, antibody (mainly immunoglobin G), and complement C3.

47. Relatively more common among Chinese of Southeast Asia (Ridley, 1985).

48. With collagen-bound immunoglobin and complement. Dermal connective tissue involvement is particularly common in certain parts of Papua and New Guinea, and occasionally elsewhere (Ridley, 1985).

49. First described by Lucio and Alverez in 1852; Latapi and Zamora, 1948; Ortiz and Giner, 1978 (reported by Pfaltzgraff and Bryceson, 1985).

50. Also in about 10% of PM (LL) form of the disease after treatment, as remarked by Ridley (1985).

51. Probably predisposed by successful chemotherapy in an interpolar or borderline patient (Ridley, 1985).

52. Not to be confused with PM (LL) vacuoles since, moreover, they contain no AFB and are not present unless there is much extracellular edema (Ridley, 1985).

References

Berhan, T.Y. Neural Leprosy—with Unusual Presentation. *Int. J. Lep.* 57(1989); Anstr. Cong. Pprs. PO 487:391.

Bharadwaj, V.P. et al. Immuno-epidemiological Studies on Sub-clinical Leprosy. *Int. J. Lep.* 57 (1989); Abstr. Cong. Pprs. FP 133: 320.

Bloom, B.R. and Mehra, V. Immunological Unresponsiveness in Leprosy. *Imm. Rev.* 80 (1984): 5–26.

Boddingius, J. Mechanisms of Nerve Damage in Leprosy. Europ. Lep. Symp., Genoa, 1981, Hlth. Coop. Pprs. I (1982): 65–84.

Bryceson, A.D.M. and Pfaltzgraff, R.E. In *Leprosy.* Ed. R.C. Hastings (Churchill Livingstone, 1985).

Dhople, A.M. Current Status and Prospects of Culture of "Mycobacterium leprae." Proc. Europ. Symp. on Lep. Res., Genoa, 1986, Hlth. Coop. Pprs. 7(1988): 9–18.

Draper, P. Structure of "Mycobacterium leprae." *Lep. Rev.* 57(1986), Supp. 2: 15–20.

Fleury, R. and Bacchi, C.E. S-100 Protein and Immuno-peroxidase as an Acid in the Histopathologic Diagnosis of Leprosy. *Int'l J. Lep.* 55(1987), 2: 338–344.

Goihman-Yar, M. Thoughts on the Immunology of Leprosy. *Int. J. Lep.* 48(1980): 435–439.

Godal, T. Leprosy Immunology—Some Aspects of the Role of the Immune System in the Pathogenesis of Disease. *Lep. Rev.* 55(1985): 407–414.

Harboe, M. The Immunology of Leprosy. In *Leprosy.* Ed. R.C. Hastings (Churchill Livingstone, 1985): 53–87.

Haregewoin, A. Investigation into T Cell Responses in Leprosy with Special Emphasis on the Immunological Unresponsiveness of Lepromatous Leprosy. Oslo, 1985, A.H.R.I., Addis Ababa and Lab. for Imm., Norsk Hydro's Inst. for Cancer Res. and the Norwegian Radium Hosp.

Hasting, R.C. Editorials. *Int. J. Lep.* 56(1988) 62–100.

Job, C.K. Transmission of Leprosy
———. Current Lit. *Int. J. Lep.* 56(1988): 147. Idem, Nerve Damage in Leprosy. *Int. J. Lpr.* 57(1989): 532–539.

Jopling, W.H. *Handbook of Leprosy*, 3rd Ed. William Heinemann, 1984.

Kato, L. A Multifactor Solid Medium for In Vitro Cultivation of "Mycobacterium leprae" and Monoclonal Antibodies. Proc. Europ. Symp. on Lep., Genoa, 1986, Hlth. Coop. Pprs. 7(1988): 9–18.

Kaufmann et al. The Social Dimension of Leprosy. ILEP, 3rd. Ed., 1986.

Languillon, J. *Precis de Leprologie* (2nd Ed., Masson, Paris, 1986.)

Liu Tze-Chun et al. Histology of Indeterminate Leprosy. *Int. J. Lep.* 50(1982): 172–176.

Mshana R,N, and Nilsen, R. Leprosy: the Immunologist and the Patient. Editorials. *Int. J. Lep.* 56(1988) 314–322.

Machin, M. A Possible Mode of Entry to the Body of "Mycobacterium leprae." *Lep. Rev.* 59(1988): 87–89.

Maier, M. The Relation between Allergy and Immunity in Leprosy. *Int. J. Lep.* 55(1987) 116–139.

Mathur, D. et al. Site of Early Lesions in Leprosy. *Int. J. Lep.* 57(1989) Anstr. Cong. Pprs. FP 017:306.

McDougall, A.C.M. and Yamalkar, S.J. Leprosy: Basic Information and Management. Ciba-Geigy, 1987.

Narayanan, R.B. et al. Immunopathology of Leprosy Granulomas—Current Status: A Review. *Lap. Rev.* 59(1988): 75–82.

Pettit, J.H.S. Should Indeterminate Leprosy Ever Be Diagnosed? *Int'l J. Lep.* 49(1981): 95–96.

Pfaltzgraff, R.E. The Management of Reactions in Leprosy. Clinical Notes. *Int. J. Lep.* 57(1989): 103–109.

Pfaltzgraff, R.E. and Bryceson, A.D.M. Clinical Leprosy. In *Leprosy.* Ed. R.C. Hastings (Churchill Livingstone, 1985): 134–176.

Rea, T.H. and Modlin, R.L. Identification of Sub-populations of CD 4 + and CD 8 + T-cells in Leprosy Granulomas. *Int. J. Lep.* (1989); Abstr. Cong. Pprs. FP 118:327.

Rees, R.J.W. The Microbiology of Leprosy. In *Leprosy.* Ed. R.C. Hastings (Churchill Livingstone, 1985): 31–52.

Reich, C.V. Leprosy: Cause, Transmission, and a New Theory of Pathogenesis. Author's Abstr., *Int. J. Lep.* 55(1987): 738.

Ridley, D.R. Skin Biopsy in Leprosy: Histological Interpretation and Clinical Application. Documents Geigy, 2nd. Ed. 1985.

Ridley, D.H. and Job, C.K. The Pathology of Leprosy. In *Leprosy.* Ed. R.C. Hastings (Churchill Livingstone, 1985): 100–133.

Samuel, N.M. et al. Ultrastructure of Human Foetal Schwann Cells in Tissue Culture Infected with "Mycobacterium leprae." *Lep. Rev.* 59(1988) 17–24.

Scollard, D.M. et al. Intralesional Cellular and Soluble Immuno-regulatory Events in Type I (Reversal) Reaction. *Int'l J. Lep.* (1989); Abstrc. Cong. Pprs. FP 046:312.

Stoner, G.L. Hypothesis: Do Phases of Immuno-suppression During a "M. leprae," Infection Determine the Leprosy Spectrum? *Lep. Rev.* 52(1981): 1–10.

Van Hoorhis, W.C. et al. The Cutaneous Infiltrates of Leprosy. *New Eng. J. Med.* 307(1982), 26:1593–1597.

Waters, M.F.R. Leprosy. *Medicine International.* Oct. 1988.

Young, D.B. Current Status of Research on Antigens of "M. leprae" and Monoclonal Antibodies. Proc. Europ. Symp. on Lep. Res., Genoa, 1986, Hlth. Coop. Pprs. 7(1988): 9–18.

The Essential Reality of the Disease

> "Leprosy is primarily a peripheral neuropathy, the manifestations of which being a polyneuritis with its classical features of motor, sensory, and trophic disorders brought about by nerve damage attributable to the affinity of 'Mycobacterium leprae' for Schwann cells"[1,2]

Fairly soon after the identification of the causative organism by Hansen, it was suggested by Virchow that peripheral nerves could, on the basis of histological findings, be the initial site of infection of the disease (Boillot, 1985). About a century later, Khanolkar held the undisproved view that all Hansen's disease is neutral in its inception (Ridley and Job, 1985). Nowadays, it is acknowledged that, as an infection, the disease has its roots only in Schwann cells of the peripheral nerves. In other words: (i) it has been validated that peripheral nerve involvement is fundamental to the establishment of infection by Hansen's bacillus (*M. leprae*); (ii) the most clinically important tissue damage in the disease is the peripheral nerve; (iii) the sequence of events starts from incipient infection from Schwann cell as the target organ of the invading organism to overt manifestation of the disease or, as previously intimated, the first step in the inception of a skin lesion is via the presence of the organism in a nerve bundle. In this respect, nerve lesions precede skin lesions by as much as five years (Browne, 1984), nerve dysfunction in the interpolar or borderline group by months or even years (Jopling, 1984). In short, even though cutaneous manifestation becomes apparent in the first place in Hansen's disease, the latter remains primarily a peripheral neuropathy the nature of which is reportedly not fully understood.

Further evidence in the light of the foregoing shows that:

- The peripheral nerve serves as an immunologically protected site to Hansen's bacillus (*M. leprae*), or acts as a immunological barrier, yet it is in the nerve that the bacillus attains a higher density than in the skin, its antigen not readily detectable therein (Ridley et al., 1986).

- Peripheral nerve rather than skin lesion is more important in assessing the real bacterial and immunological status of the hansenian (leprosy patient), even though this is not a practical proposition on a routine basis, as has been pointed out.

- The finding of an immunological granuloma or a bacilli in the nerve is more significant than cellular infiltrate alone, and in the nerve it is diagnostic of the disease as has been reported.

- Upon involvement of the nerve held in check by immune mechanisms, there is no resulting skin lesion.

- Hansen's disease is the most common cause of peripheral neuropathy and, as a result, the most crippling of diseases. By the same token, the disease is the third most important cause of blindness worldwide.

- Sensory loss or insensitivity as a result of nerve involvement is the most insidious and foremost complication of the disease, the main factor predisposing to secondary infection, the major mediator of disability and/or deformity, as has been expressed.

- Whereas disability and/or deformity is the ultimate, more important, event in a sequence not yielding all the answers, it sets the disease apart from other diseases in the eyes of the lay person, as remarked by Brand and Fritschi (1985).

- The occurrence of disability and/or deformity in a given endemic area might prove a more reliable index of control of the disease than its very incidence (Smith et al., 1980).

- The single most important aspect of the management of Hansen's disease is the prevention of nerve damage, prevention of the development of associated disability and/or deformity being one of the three objectives for control purposes, as has been emphasized.

- Not halting or reversing the sequelae of nerve damage in time merely accentuates an otherwise adverse impact on both patient and community alike from a psychological and socioeconomic standpoint, as well recognized.

Hallmarks of a Common Fate

The bite of Hansen's disease lies in peripheral
neuropathy and its sequelae.[3]

As already intimated, nerve lesions precede skin lesions in an
appreciable way, an early manifestation in polar paucibacillary (PP)
or TT form of the disease, a late one in the polar multibacillary (PM)
or LL form. While it is not clear whether impaired blood vessels (cf.
the blood-nerve barrier) and the impaired perineurial function (cf. the
perineurial barrier) in Hansen's disease imply cause or consequence
of neuropathy, as expressed by Shetty and Antia (1988), this
neuropathy can, incidentally, manifest itself in both patients and their
contacts without any clinical evidence, i.e., as an insidious "quiet nerve
paralysis" or silent neuritis, a reportedly more common phenomenon
than previously suspected.

Either way, the overall picture testifies to a common fate shared
by the two polar forms and the borderline group of the disease if not
checked in time: disability and/or deformity.

It has been mentioned that predilection of Hansen's bacillus (*M.
leprae*)—or its affinity—for Schwann cells reported by Weddell et al.
in 1963[4] has run out of favor since these cells are now thought of as,
instead, host cells to the pathogen by providing its protection (Boddingius, 1982; Ridley, 1985; Ridley et al. 1986). What is of immediate
interest as regards the organism is its primary entry into the peripheral
nerve.

The mode of entry of Hansen's bacillus (*M. leprae*) and dissemination with in the peripheral nerve brings in a variety of views:
intra-axonal transport of the bacillus suggested by Khanolkar (1963),
Schwannian relay via endoneurial blood vessels proposed by Jopling
(1984) and others,[5] retrograde, intra-Schwannian or intra-macrophage routes from dermal nerve endings forwarded by Boddingius
(1982), in respect, mostly, of transmission.

Credit for the elaboration of mode(s) of entry of the bacillus goes
to Job (1989), who outlines four possibilities: (i) through naked dermal
filaments in the epidermis and spread centripetally (upstream) along
the axon, albeit that intra-axonal bacilli are rarely found there; (ii)
phagocytosis of the bacilli by Schwann cells in the upper dermis and

dissemination by contiguity; (iii) bacilli initially taken up by macrophages in the upper dermis around adnexae of the skin and nerve bundles, ingested by perineurial cells following their release from macrophages, and passed on to Schwann cells (alternatively, bacilli-loaded macrophages infiltrate the perineurium and invade the nerve); (iv) through the blood circulation via intraneural capillaries as perhaps the most frequent route of entry, on the plea that bacillemia is common to all forms of Hansen's disease.

Whether peripheral nerve involvement is early[6] or late phenomenon (Boddingius, 1982), or sensory (unmyelinated) fibers affected[7] or rather motor (myelinated) fibers, remain open questions. Of more relevant importance at the moment is the nature of nerve damage.

The Roots of Damage

> "A proper understanding of the mechanism(s) of nerve damage in leprosy is of paramount importance in the prevention, treatment, and modulation of damage itself."

Views on the mechanism(s) of damage to peripheral nerves in Hansen's disease remain diverse, unclear, and not satisfactorily understood, as has been noticed elsewhere, in that linked in part to the absence of suitable animal models, and the fact that the histological picture is distinct in the two polar forms of the disease, thus raising the possibility that different mechanisms might be involved from the start.

Either way, one is reminded by Antia et al. (1989) that the above views rest on studies on nerves at a late active stage of the disease invariably associated with the presence of inflammation. Moreover, the authors have, over the years, gathered enough substantial evidence that early changes in hansenic (leprous) nerves can occur in the absence of either inflammatory cells or overt presence of antigens.

As regards the roots of nerve damage, one ought to distinguish between causes and factors attributable to, or associated with, them, in keeping with the various forms of the disease. Thus:

Causes specific to the polar paucibacillary (PP) or TT and border-line group

Nerve damage, as the common denominator of the above forms of disease, reaches its peak in the borderline paucibacillary (BP) or BT, as already intimated, and is not the direct result of infection, rather, as acknowledged by now, the consequence of immunological reaction to antigenic elements liberated from Hansen's bacillus (*M. leprae*) in and around peripheral nerves, as remarked by Bloom and Mehra (1984), hence more appropriately referred to as immunological damage to nerves. Godal (1984) elaborates the point further, in that the host's attack on the bacillus within the nerves—as evidenced by the presence of the immulogical granuloma mostly in PP (TT) and BP (BT) forms—leading to the killing of the pathogen by activated macrophages, extorts a price: distortion and damage of nerve fibers, particularly more pronounced in immunologically-mediated complications (viz. "reversal" of Jopling's Type I reaction) whereby a rapid build-up of immunological attack on the pathogen in the case.

While advocating the necessity to make clear distinction between sensory and motor nerve damage, Mshana et al. (1980) express the view that two different mechanisms are involved:

(i) An immune granulomatous reaction (viz. immunological granuloma) secondary to interaction between Hansen's bacillus (*M. leprae*) and Schwann cells of unmyelinated sensory fibers leading to the triad sensory loss, hypopigmentation, and hair loss.

(ii) A consequence of delayed hypersensitivity (DHR) to intraneural antigens liberated from the pathogen affecting motor or major nerve trunks.

Causes specific to the polar multibacillary (PM) or LL form of the disease

Via an unrestricted multiplication of the pathogen in Schwann cells, perineurial cells, and macrophages in and around peripheral nerves leading to a slow, insidious destruction of nerves (in years) by way of perineurial fibroses and hyalinization of the nerve parenchyma as reported by Job (1989).

Factors involved in all forms of the disease

There are four factors, in the opinion of Job (1989), worthy of consideration:

(i) Cooler sites of the peripheral nerve helping bacterial localization and multiplication; (ii) trauma to those peripheral nerve trunks usually superficially placed; (iii) increase in intraneural pressure; (iv) occlusive changes of intraneural blood vessels.

It has also been suggested that continuing nerve damage following infection with Hansen's bacillus (*M. leprae*) may be associated with degraded bacterial antigens and non-acid stage in the life style cycle of the pathogen.

What Statistics Cannot Convey

> Disability and/or deformity follow the inexorable law of expected consequences when, either way, steps are not taken in their favor in time.

The sheer perpetuation of disability and/or deformity in Hansen's disease testifies if nothing else to a combination of obduracy and inadequacy unmatched by any other incapacitating condition, so much so that it has been rightly said that the disease is disability and/or deformity unable to be measured psychologically and socioeconomically.

As is the case with statistics relating to the true prevalence of the disease worldwide, information on the corresponding status of disability and/or deformity is wanting or, when at hand, not comparable as a rule.

While treatment at present covers but one out of every five or four hansenians (leprosy patients) in endemic areas, Bechelli and Ruffino-Netto (1985) are of the opinion that "of the total estimated number of patients (10,786,000) in the world, 3,870,000 could have disabilities." This alarming enough figure —almost certainly on the increase since then—reflects quite a global problem, in that, as admitted in the report from the 1988 Congress Workshop on Prevention and Management of Impairment in Leprosy, control programs over the world have not succeeded in mastering the existence of disability and/or deformity.

The magnitude of the problem entails a dimension less of physical restriction or ungainly sight than loss of human dignity and suffering that no statistical evidence can impart, let alone the considerable financial burden imposed on society. While, in this respect, one could without irony refer to the banal authority of disability and/or deformity, there is of late a disturbing report that regularity of treatment with dapsone may be associated with the condition (Hasting, 1987).

It would seem that the true significance of disability and/or deformity in Hansen's disease is reflected by lack of awareness, emphasis, or commitment at appropriate levels where responsibility lies, as has been inferred. To put it more bluntly, the problem is compounded of (i) lack of early diagnosis of the disease and of early recognition of nerve damage by appropriate yet practical methods; (ii) inadequate therapeutic measures; (iii) absence of instructions to the patient or patient's self-neglect; (iv) insufficient or nonexistent health education with the help of the media; and (v) professional indifference and social apathy.

In this context, it is fair to add that the psychological or stigmatizing import of deformity as such, and even worse, mutilation, comes into it, in that authors like Brand (1981) and Brand and Fritschi (1985) are of the opinion that the loathesomeness and fear of Hansen's disease are rooted in its physical handicap to the point that the very mention of the word "leprosy" conjures up the manifold aspects of the handicap, a view, incidentally, queried by Warren (1972) to the contrary.

A Predictable Pattern of Involvement

> Peripheral nerves, immune as a rule to bacillary invasion, find one single exception with Hansen's bacillus (*M. leprae*), as has been observed.

Experience has it that, if coped with in time, nerve damage is reversible. Reason tells us that it is much more important to recognize mild (early) nerve damage, which stands a good chance of recovery with appropriate therapeutic measures. Either way, only specific peripheral nerves are affected in Hansen's disease, upon the well-established postulates that (i) sites of predilection lie superficially and thus cooler, the bacillus having, besides, affinity for temperature lower than body temperature; (ii) the nerves involved, by virtue of their very anatomical position, are more vulnerable and hence liable to trauma; (iii) constant tugging on those nerves through movement accentuates damage usually proximal to the joint.

Cutaneous (sensory) nerves

It is essential to distinguish clearly between cutaneous or sensory nerve damage and damage affecting major (motor) nerve trunks, in that while the latter is more obvious clinically by virtue of its visual impact, sensory loss or insensitivity to pain of hands and feet—or absence of warning function of pain sensation—equates a lack of warning system that makes the hansenian (leprosy patient) prone to accidental injuries of any kind, as remarked by Rolston and Chesteen (1970).

Whereas the major importance of Hansen's disease stems from nerve damage it provokes, sensory loss or insensitivity is much more far reaching than considered as a mere prelude to disability and/or deformity: it is the acknowledged earliest and most severely affected modality of nerve damage, the tip of the iceberg, as observed by Lechat (1981).

Let it be recalled that loss of tactile sensation or lack of recognition of touch entails a dissociation between the hansenian's (leprosy patient's) affected part(s) of his body and "self," as has been pointed out: these two co-exist no more, the former extending beyond the limits of the latter, thus explaining the propensity of the patient not to react normally to the occurrence of superimposed injuries to his insensitive limb(s). Sensory impairment is an early manifestation of the PP (TT) form of Hansen's disease, as has been intimated, and whereby, bacilli are scanty or absent, and cutaneous nerves harboring these organisms show evidence of granulomatous infiltration, i.e., immunological granuloma. By contrast, PM (LL) form of the disease, while harboring very large numbers of bacilli, develops sensory loss or insensitivity late in the disease.

Major (motor) nerve trunks

Involvement of major (motor) nerve trunks in Hansen's disease follows an order of frequency, more so, as has been intimated previously, in the advent of immunological complications or reactions ("reversal" or Jopling's Type I) met in the BP (BT) form of the disease. Thus:

(i) Ulnar nerve: weakness in fourth and fifth fingers and wasting of interossei muscles. Impaired sensation in ulnar border of hand. **[Claw Hand]**

(ii) Median nerve: weakness of the thumb and wasting of its muscles. Impaired sensation of the palm of the hand.

(iii) Facial (seventh cranial) nerve: Weakness of eyelids (lagophthalmos) and of facial muscles (facial paresis or palsy). If not treated, ultimately blindness.

(iv) Lateral popliteal or common peroneal nerve: foot drop.

(v) Posterior tibial nerve: claw toes and impaired sensation of the sole of the foot.

(vi) Radial nerve: wrist drop.

(vii) Fifth cranial nerve: ocular pathology.

(viii) Great auticular nerve: usually symptomless.

(ix) Cervical nerve: usually symptomless.

(x) Supraorbital nerve: usually symptomless, too.

Concerning the various forms of Hansen's disease, Brand and Fritschi (1985) summarized the respective pattern of nerve damage pertaining to these clinical forms as follows:

Polar paucibacilliary (PP) or TT form

Rapid early total sensory loss confined to patches of involved skin, followed by neuritis spreading proximally along sensory to mixed nerves. Marked localized swelling of nerves. Occasional caseation and nerve abscess formation. Sudden paralysis sometimes due to uninvolved nerve bundles becoming compressed in the same sheath with involved bundle.

Polar multibacillary (PM) or LL form

Slow development of temperature-dependent patterns of sensory loss confined to the surface layers, followed, years later, by a superimposed pattern of motor and deep sensory loss based on damage to mixed nerve trunks which lie in cool superficial sites. The quiet progressive nerve damage may be suddenly interrupted and exacerbated by acute neuritis caused by inflammatory swelling of nerves in tight sheaths and in tight canals causing entrapment.

Interpolar or borderline group

Mixture of features of the above polar forms. The combination of the widespread nature of many borderline cases with the more active immune response results sometimes in very severe nerve damage in all four limbs and face.

The Ongoing Process

> Disability and/or deformity is neither an ineluc-
> table fact of Hansen's disease nor an ines-
> capable issue: it need not, and ought not, be the
> case in the advent of preventive measures.

To state that disability and/or deformity in Hansen's disease adds up to the status of the patient would be beside the point: it is before anything else an all too familiar, perennial sight associated with fatalistic undertones, an essential component of the disease as viewed by the layman.

While the hansenian (leprosy patient) is paying an additional price for his disability and/or deformity, fear, aversion, repulsion—and similar reactions from the public at large and society in particular—stem from precisely the negative visual impact of such physical impairment, rather from the accentuation of that impact itself.

Either way, the situation is at the expense of what is more realistically at stake: a preventable event that is, instead, allowed to pursue its tragic outcome. In other words, the pathways from nerve damage to sensory loss and motor nerve deficit have been—and still are—paved with neglect of one kind or other.

Admittedly, many patients with disability and/or deformity first report for treatment when nerve damage has already set in, or is too far gone, i.e, irreversibly so. Whether through ignorance and/or neglect, which top the list of possible causes, non-availability of medical care, or, when at hand, inadequacy of treatment and/or follow-up ought to be added to it. Branbsma (1981) mentions equally undetectable early neuritis.

At this juncture, the loose and, moreover, indiscriminate use of the terms disability and deformity in the literature calls for a timely clarification, if not correction.

From a neurological standpoint, disability means a deficit of function (physiological); deformity, a structural deviation from the norm (anatomical). In short, in Hansen's disease, disability is sensory deprival or deprivation (cf. tactile sensation, temperature, and pain); deformity, alteration or modification of shape and function leading, if not checked in time, to mutilation.

What is more, disability and deformity as such are the exception, their interrelatedness the rule as illustrated in the chart on the following page.

The above suggests that, in order to avoid imprecision or confusion: (i) the term disability be solely applied to sensory loss per se, as well as its ocular sequelae; (ii) the term deformity implying either deformity as such or its interrelatedness with disability other than ocular pathology; (iii) the term disability and/or deformity be used in a general sense.

The Tortured Architecture

> "Time lost in early recognition of nerve damage means ignored years of grace."

Disability and/or deformity appertains mostly to endemic areas of the Third World, yet bears witness to what is not being currently achieved: general awareness of the problem, recognition of the early neural involvement, and appropriate countermeasures.

Spectrum of Disability and Deformity in Hansen's Disease

	Feature	Modality	Disability	Deformity	Interrelatedness
FACE	Madarosis	a		+	
	Lagophthalmos	s/m		+	
	Loss of corneal reflex	s	+		
	Synechiae	s	+		
	Keratitis	s	+		
	Blurred vision	s	+		
	Blindness	s	+		
	Facial palsy	s/m			+
	Leonine facies			+	
	Hoarse voice			+	
	Collapse of nose			+	
	Gynaecomastia			+	
HAND	Sensory loss		+		
	Ulceration	a/s			+
	Wasting of thenar and hypothenar emniences	a/s/m			+
	Contraction (fingers not ankylosed)	a/s/m			+
	Claw hand	a/s/m			+
	Wrist drop	a/s/m			+
	Absorption of digits	a/s/m			+
FOOT	Sensory loss	s	+		
	Clawing of toes	a/s/m			+
	Foot drop	a/s/m			+
	Plantar ulceration	a/s			+
	Absorption of toes	a/s/m			+

a = autonomic
s = sensory
m = motor

This multifactorial state of affairs calls for a deeper insight into the pathogenesis of disability and/or deformity since, as has been intimated beforehand, (i) the single most important aspect of the management of Hansen's disease is the prevention of neural involvement and its sequelae; and (ii) not halting or reversing that situation in time would merely accentuate an otherwise adverse impact on both patient and community from a psychological and socioeconomic standpoint, perhaps, more philosophically, because in terms of prevention, "Seldom does such a neglected disease give such a long warning. Seldom is such a clear warning so sadly disregarded."[8]

While the urgency of the problem is emphasized enough in the literature, and accorded by the responsible authorities the attention it deserves, central to one's appreciation of the pathogenesis of disability and/or deformity in Hansen's disease is the chart on the next page, inspired from Bryceson and Pfaltzgraff's (1979).

It can be seen to what an extent sensory loss or insensitivity is the most important cause of damage, bearing in mind, though, that the similar end results are met in diabetes, tabes dorsalis, and spina bifida. In the same vein, minor injuries are potential major disasters, as has been stressed, which led Brand and Fritschi (1985) to formulate primary deformity as being due directly to Hansen's disease, and secondary deformity through the patient's self negligence, hence occurring as a result of the primary problem.

Plantar or trophic ulceration is possibly the commonest secondary complication of the disease, as is well known to those with experience of it.

Bone damage also occurs as a result of direct infiltration of Hansen's bacillus (*M. leprae*) in the PM (LL) form of the disease.

The Wages of Neglect

> "Knowing when and how to intervene during a disease process is as important as—perhaps more important—than curing that disease."

The rapidly changing areas of medicine are strewn correspondingly with new challenges. Life sciences are being explored further

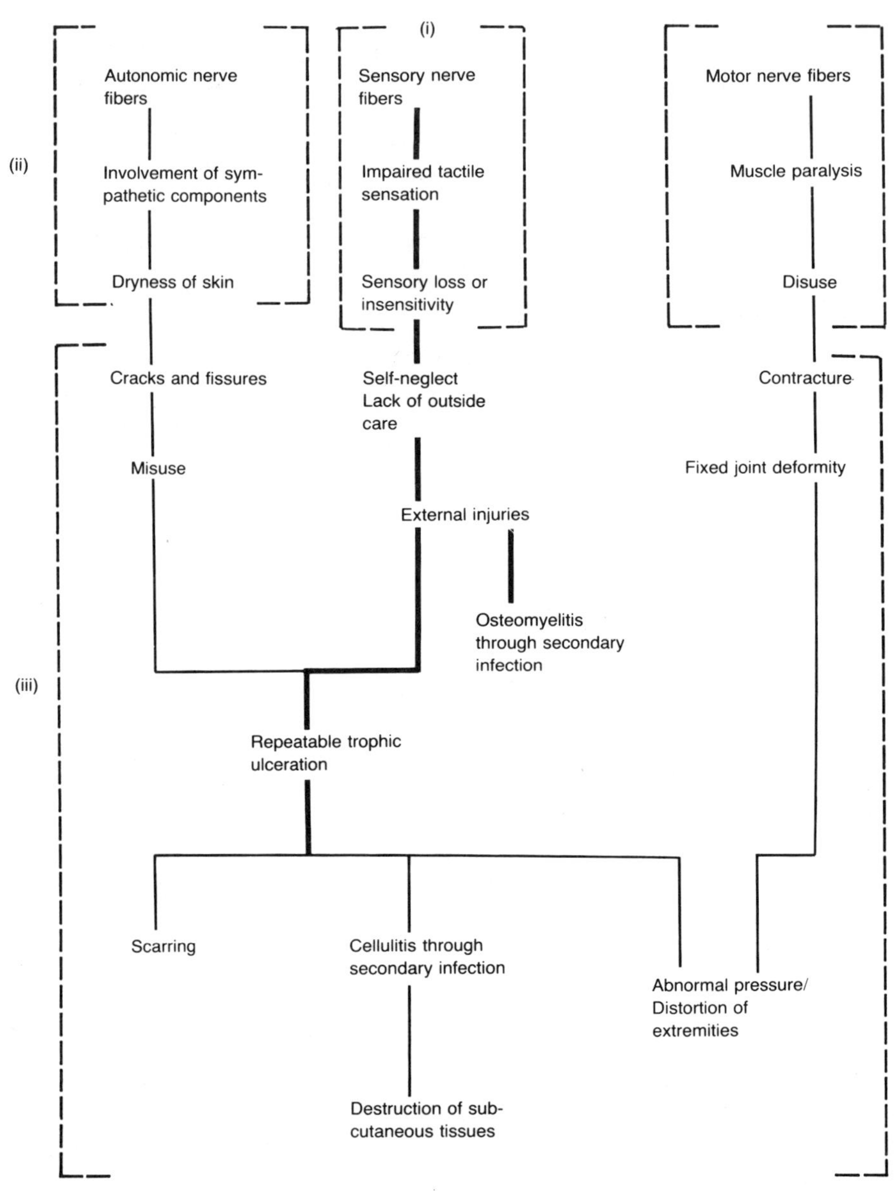

(ii)
Autonomic nerve fibers
Involvement of sympathetic components
Dryness of skin
Cracks and fissures
Misuse

(i)
Sensory nerve fibers
Impaired tactile sensation
Sensory loss or insensitivity
Self-neglect Lack of outside care
External injuries
Osteomyelitis through secondary infection

Motor nerve fibers
Muscle paralysis
Disuse
Contracture
Fixed joint deformity

(iii)
Repeatable trophic ulceration
Scarring
Cellulitis through secondary infection
Destruction of subcutaneous tissues
Abnormal pressure/ Distortion of extremities

(i) Disability
(i) + (ii) Primary nerve damage
(iii) Sequelae

afield, most of them already hints of tomorrow in our affluent and cultish Western societies, yet with the notable exception of those Third World countries where poverty, malnutrition, infectious and parasitic disease overshadow the other problems as has been altogether remarked. Hansen's disease, as the most common crippling condition, is proving no exception to this.

One reason, as regards the less privileged countries, is that the gap between front line attacks on those very problems and the means available to overcome them is not closing. Far from it. Another, perhaps more important, reason is that the old adage that one ounce of prevention is better that one pound of cure has not penetrated collective health strategies, nor triggered a shift of emphasis in health thinking within the responsible structures.

Traditional one-sided curative medicine, not primary or preventive health care, wins the day in the wake of avoidable suffering, as has been pointed out.[9]

Converting professional and lay collectivities to the evidence that, by a long shot, prevention is better than cure is one of the most arduous tasks of health education at all levels. As has been intimated, it is less a question of preventionism than a re-adaption to the demands of a situation that begs the obvious: recasting one's mind to the necessity of preventive measures as a top priority—without neglecting any clinical coverage of the sick—means being more a keeper of health than dispenser of drugs to patients.[10]

The possibilities of prevention of Hansen's disease is best illustrated by means of several levels of intervention during the disease process. Thus:

The following diagram calls for these comments:

- Level 1 or primary intervention: intervening at this level is not possible at this stage owing to a lack of appropriate immuno-epidemiological tools (viz. immunodiagnosis and immunoprophylaxis) that would intervene between exposure and onset of disease while at the same time protecting the populations at risk. Much more is to be achieved before the sort of intervention proves technically and economically sound, and applicable to field conditions. However remote at the moment the implementation of such a program, it is at this level, and this level alone, that

Levels of intervention in Hansen's Disease

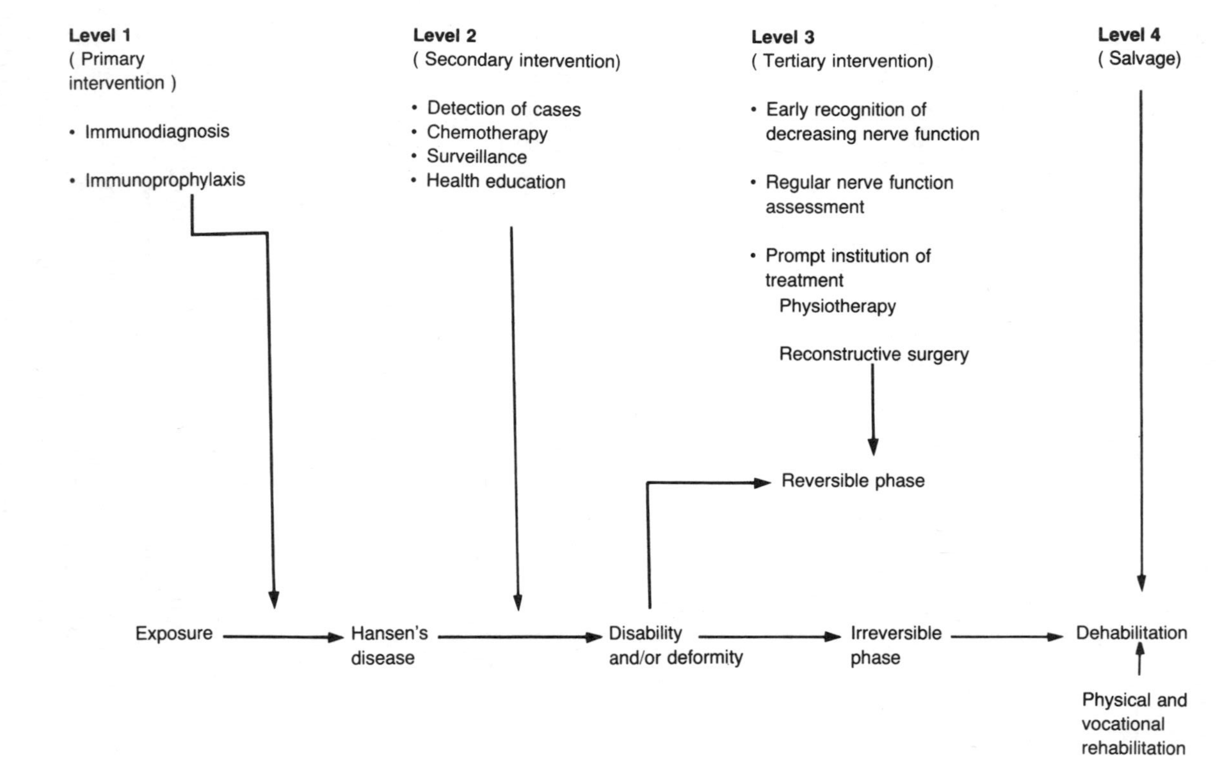

eventual eradication of Hansen's disease could take place by stopping the transmission process.

- Level 2 or secondary intervention embodies the next logical step which, properly coped with, could ward off the onset of disability and or deformity.

  Yet judging by the increasing incidence of physical handicap or crippling incurred by the disease mostly in Third World countries, this level sticks to its reputation as being the bane of control, presumably on account of (i) patients keeping in hiding still, (ii) inadequate case detection, (iii) insufficient therapeutic coverage, (iv) poor or nonexistent recognition and/or assessment of nerve damage, (v) absence of surveillance, and (vi) ineffective health education.

- Level 3 or tertiary intervention: this highly selective level applies to a restricted number of institutions worldwide, able to afford such remedial measures in the hands of skilled professional staff and personnel, a most praiseworthy endeavor unfortunately reserved for the chosen few.

- Level 4 or salvage is by no means something of the past. As an irreversible phase up to mutilations, it reflects the epitome of neglect from whatever cause, the utter failure of the human factor. Salvage means when and where it can be carried out.

Notes

1. Reference to neural involvement in Hansen's disease is quite a later recognition in the annals of medicine, as has been remarked: it came to attention in Danielssen and Boeck's work in 1847.
2. WHO Study Group on Peripheral Neuropathy, 1980.
3. C.f. "The bite of the disease lies in the disability it causes, and this is mainly a result of damage to nerve" (Hill-Smith, 1981).
4. Quoted by Hill-Smith (1981) and Boddingius (1982).
5. Dastur, Pearson, and Ross, quoted by Hill-Smith (1981).
6. Rees and Waters, quoted by Hill-Smith (1981).
7. Shetty et al., quoted by Boddingius (1982).
8. Expressed by the present writer (1967).
9. Let alone the practitioner of curative medicine defending every inch of his professional turf, as well as his purse, as has been pointed out; when too much expenditure and effort are being devoted to advanced and/or sophisticated tertiary health services; when too little primary or preventive health care is still the rule. It would thus seem that somewhere along the line, curative health care has always managed to get higher priority, in that it is probably more glamorous

to put up a modern, fully equipped hospital than combat malnutrition, help fight killer diseases, or eliminate poverty and squalor at the source, as has been similarly pointed out.

10. As that grand old man of modern medicine, Jonas Salk, puts it: "We have schools of medicine that produce doctors of medicine. Perhaps what we need are schools of health that produce doctors of health."

References

Antia, N.H. et al. Indication that Early Events Causing Nerve Damage in Leprosy May Not Be Immunologically-Mediated. *Int. J. Lpr.* 57(1989); Abstr. Cong. Pprs. FP 171: 337.

Bechelli, L.M. and Ruffino-Netto, A. Psycho-social and Economical Aspects of Leprosy and Tuberculosis. *Acta Lepr.* 3(1985)4: 295–305.

Bloom, B.R. and Mehra, V. Immunological Unresponsiveness in Leprosy. *Imm. Rev.* 80(1984): 5–28.

Boddingius, J. Mechanisms of Peripheral Nerve Damage in Leprosy. Europ. Lep. Symp., Genoa, 1981, Hlth Coop. Pprs. 1(1982):65–84.

Boillot, F. Aspects Actuels de la Neuropathie Hansenienne: A propos d'une experience de 13 mois au Senegal. These (1985) Présentée à l'Université Scientifique et Medicale de Grenoble.

Brand, P.W. and Fritschi, E.P. Rehabilitation in Leprosy. In *Leprosy.* Ed. R.C. Hastings (Churchill Livingstone, 1985):287–319.

Brandsma, W. Basic Nerve Function Assessment in Leprosy Patients. *Lep. Rev.* 52(1981):161–170.

Browne, S.G. *Leprosy.* Documenta Geigy, Acta Clinica, 1984.

Bryceson, A.D.M. and Pfaltzgraff, R.E. In *Leprosy.* 2nd Ed. (Churchill Livingstone, 1979).

Ffytche, T.J. The Eye and Leprosy. Editorial. *Lep. Rev.* 52(1981): 111–119.

Godal, T. Leprosy Immunology—Some Aspects of the Role of the Immune System in the Pathogenesis of Disease. *Lep. Rev.* 55(1984): 407–414.

Hastings, R.C. The 1986 Journal. A Continuing Perspective. *Int. J. Lep.* 55(1987): 140–156.

Hill-Smith, I. The immunopathology of Nerve Damage in Leprosy. *Int. J. Lep.* 49(1981): 223–227.

Job, C.K. Nerve Damage in Leprosy. *Int. J. Lpr.* (1989): 532–539.

Jopling, W.H. *Handbook of Leprosy.* 3rd Ed. (William Heinemann, 1984).

Khanolkar,V.R. Ciba Foundation Study Group on the Pathogenesis of Leprosy, London, 1963.

Mallac (de), M.J. Onset and Pattern of Deformity in Leprosy. *Lep. Rev.* 37(1967): 71–91.

Mshana, R.N. et al. The Immunopathology of Nerve Damage in Leprosy. *Int. J. Rep.* 50(1982): 367–368.

Pfaltzgraff, R.E. and Bryceson, A.D.M. In *Leprosy.* Ed. R.C. Hastings (Churchill Livingstone, 1985): 134–176.

Reports from Congress Workshop: Prevention and Management of Impairment in Leprosy. *Int. J. Lep.* 57(1989): 290–291.

Ridley, D.R. and Job, C.K. The Pathology of Leprosy. In *Leprosy.* Ed. R.C. Hastings (Churchill Livingstone, 1985): 100–133.

Rolston, M.A. and Chesteen, H.E. The Identification of Psychological Factors Related to the Rehabilitation of Leprosy Patients. Final Report, 1970, School of Social Welfare, Louisiana State University, Baton Rouge.

Ridley, M.J. et al. Events Surrounding the Recognition of "Mycobacterium Leprae" in Nerves. *Int. J. Lep.* 55(1986): 95–106.

Shetty, V.P. and Anita, N.H. Nerve Damage in Leprosy. Correspondence. *Int. J. Lep.* 56(1988): 619–621.

Smith, W.C.S. et al. Disability in Leprosy: a Relevant Measurement of Progress in Leprosy Control. *Lep. Rev.* 51(1980): 155–165.

Warren, A.G. Are Deformities Stigmatizing? A Surgeon's Approach. *Lep. Rev.* 43(1972): 74–82.

The Channels of Control

> The ultimate test of a control program's intentions is not its rhetoric, but the specific action it is taking towards achieving a realistic and cost-effective goal based on both bold and innovative approaches, hence bridging the gap between principles and practice of that control.

It is sobering to reflect that at the levels of health care delivery system there is seemingly no integrated philosophy equating global planning with execution, concerted resolution with commitment, or overall strategy with deed. Instead, a cleavage exist whereby the call for initiative from the top is not being equally matched by the response to it from below.

Be it as it may. The elimination of most communicative diseases from First World countries took place long before drugs and vaccines were available for the control, writes Antia (1982). In the view of the author:

> Education combined with improvement of the social and economic conditions thereof remaining the only certain way of controlling communicable diseases. They are more amenable to social and political action rather than purely medical measures.

While acknowledging that science has not the answer to most human problems, Antia concedes that, with the exception of smallpox, the causes of failure to control communicable diseases of Third World countries are attributable to:

> Inadequate funds, non-availability of drugs, suitable personnel and transport, ignorance and apathy of the people and their rulers, and finally the development of resistance to drugs and insecticides and the non-availability or the exorbitant cost of alternative treatment.

The author's further remarks are pertinent for the unity of purpose of this chapter:

> Failure to achieve results despite vast inputs of men and money could have been condoned in the early phases as genuine lack of appreciation of these factors, but the continuation and expansion of services which have proved to be inadequate or ineffective can only be attributable to vested interest of professionals, bureaucracy, pharmaceutical industries, and politicians in propagating the empires built by them on various diseases. Any new approach, however well based on scientific and/or social reality, is firmly resisted on administrative or technical grounds. . . . In the poor and chiefly rural societies of developing countries this implies that decisions are made by a small coterie of the urban elite, who, even if well intentioned, have little concept of the actual problems of the majority of the people with whom they have little physical and cultural affinity.

In fact, as has been expressed elsewhere, most Third World countries still rely on the upkeep of external technical and scientific help or guidance, support for the implementation and extension of their control programs additional mobilization and coordination of material resources towards training, health education, rehabilitation, etc. Yet "in many developing countries the basic resources are insufficient, and it is difficult to make rapid progress with a larger allocation and international cooperation."[1]

These countries, in turn, are encouraged or even urged to step up their control programs through integrated health services, or existing primary health care (PHC) units: strengthen health education at community level; provide more facilities for the multidisciplinary training of para-medical personnel; improve the quality of case-finding, diagnosis, and therapeutic coverage; enforce health education; promote rehabilitation; and ensure the legal rights of the patients, etc., as has been altogether emphasized by WHO.

Inequities in health involve gross differences which still prevail in many Third World countries—as in some First World areas—notwithstanding that "both developed and developing countries frequently fail to make efficient use of the resources that are assigned for health purposes." Besides, it ought to be borne in mind that in this context:

(i) Only a fraction of the total global biomedical research effort is being devoted to diseases from which two thirds of the Third World populations suffer. Godal estimated about 1% in 1978.

(ii) The demographic explosion or population juggernaut in the poorest Third World countries—apart from being the most urgent and pressing socioeconomic problem of our times—implies a corresponding increase of populations exposed to communicable diseases, hence of the patients. Hansen's disease is, once more, proving no exception to it.

(iii) An estimate of over 80% of the rural, slum-dwelling, and nomadic people has no access to adequate health services (Buchmann, 1982).

In the case of Hansen's disease, organized efforts at controlling it took place in the early fifties, and while it is gratifying to hear of the increasing role of non-governmental organizations in the control of the disease, the significant progress of multidrug therapy (MDT), and the promising research directed at the development of immunodiagnostic and immuno-prophylactic tools, there are further considerations to be taken into account. Thus:

(i) The disease—probably due to its particular aura—is intrinsically more difficult to cope with at an integrated health services level, as has been pointed out, hence embodying a global challenge over decades to come.

(ii) International and private organizations dedicated to Hansen's disease in all its aspects have, in spite of their very valuable investment, to reckon with political uncertainties, gross economic instability, or open hostility directed at Western religious missions, as has been mentioned elsewhere.

(iii) Most authorities involved in the control of the disease reportedly fail to consider the all-important social and psychological factors, as well as cultural, racial, and religious differences liable to be altogether quite useful in the approach, care, and treatment of the patients.

Lessons at Hand

> Unless the shortcomings inherent in the control
> of Hansen's disease in a given area come out in
> the open, and are critically assessed, and
> remedied, the way ahead would be jeopardized
> still.

It would be advisable to have a closer look at the multifaceted problems that beset the control of Hansen's disease since, as already intimated, despite an abundance of goodwill and dedication, laudable and worthwhile efforts from all quarters, (i) there has been no breakthrough of the overall control program of the disease; and (ii) there is no evidence that the disease (viz. its prevalence) is declining worldwide, the ensuing prospects of its eradication in view of the present available resources and methodology even more remote. Thus:

- Not being a "killer" disease, Hansen's disease hasn't the same appeal as, for instance, tuberculosis, cancer, or AIDS. It is, instead, regarded by health planners as "an apparently complex and unrewarding disease whose chronic nature and the slow effect of its chemotherapy requires long term action and hence substantial resources committed over extended period" (Buchmann, 1982).

- The disease remains to a large extent the legacy of the poor and destitute with its trail of overcrowding, promiscuity, incorrect eating habits, malnutrition, poor hygiene, and not enough confidence in Western medicine, as has been put forward, too.

Even in Europe, in the words of Leiker (1982):

The public, the authorities and medical practitioners are not sufficiently familiar with the basic facts about the disease, too often the attitude towards the disease and towards the patient is still dominated by outdated concepts. . . . Many medical practitioners do not readily recognize the early signs of the disease and they are not familiar with its modern management. . . . The image that leprosy is always a disabling disease is maintained, with its negative effects on patients and public.

The author comes to the conclusion that "our heritage of prejudice and ignorance about leprosy is still looming among us."

It has been suggested that, even though poorly understood, nutrition and diet have a global impact on the immune system (Foster et al., 1988), yet one would tend to agree that their deleterious effect on hanesenians (leprosy patients) by way of inadequate calorie intake per day do remain, as has been remarked, a stumbling block not remedied for the control of the disease.

Another stumbling block is the wide, if not increasing, gap between high technology research and patient care in endemic areas where, according to Leiker (1982), research is not commensurate with the improvement of results as far as Hansen's disease is concerned.

- From an epidemiological viewpoint, the lack of logistical support in terms of communication, geographical isolation, roads, transport, etc. makes it difficult for the hansensians (leprosy patients) to attend the nearest health center, as well as for the paramedical staff to reach these patients, as has been remarked.

  Control of Hansen's disease is still mostly carried out by special services—government and non-government alike—limited, though, to well-defined areas. Despite untiring and devoted work at all levels concerned, the number of patients has not decreased commensurately with control measures, as has been stated.

  The predominance of secondary and tertiary prevention or epidemiological intervention is still the rule, and not primary intervention that would stop transmission of the disease at the source, as expressed by Bloom (1985), in that "the major source of transmission of leprosy is from man to man. By eliminating that very source of transmission, the potential to eliminate the disease is all there."

  The determinants that would explain (i) the long incubation period or latency of Hansen's disease, (ii) its identification and modes of transmission, and (iii) sub-clinical infection, not having been determined yet, prove major setbacks in the fight against the disease and its control, as reported by Lechat (1981).

  The prevalence rate of the disease^2 although reported to be on the decline in many endemic areas, is said not to be accompanied by a corresponding reduction in the number of new cases annually, i.e., the incidence rate of Hansen's disease being estimated at involving some three-quarter million patients. On the other hand, while patient detection is the only measure of that incidence, and case-holding for control purposes happen to be wanting on the whole, accurate data regarding the actual year of onset and duration of the disease from the patients are often unreliable, as pointed out by Shepard (1983).

Too few population surveys and the failure to apply epidemiological principles of control contribute to the non-interruption of the cycle of transmission of Hansen's disease (viz. identification of infectious patients, household and sibling contacts, specific high-risk groups with appropriate chemotherapy, surveillance, etc.), as has been reported.

Scarcity of information, poor or nonexistent notification of cases or national records—particularly in those countries where the disease might be endemic—are the acknowledged bane of any control program, in that as intimated by Zuniga (1988), the almost static global magnitude of the disease is often based on unsystematic criteria and reports.

Failure of control of Hansen's disease in the areas concerned—not as a direct result of social stigmatization—has been ascribed to patients keeping in hiding, their ignorance and/or self-neglect, indifference, or apathy linked to irregularity of treatment.

The role played by environmental factors (viz. household and sibling contacts, nutritional status, overcrowding, promiscuity, poverty, hygiene, illiteracy, ethnic variations, intercurrent infections, migration, etc.) is not being determined on a worldwide basis. In the same vein, the underprivileged being the most susceptible to infection and immuno-incompetence as a result of living conditions well below standards, opportunity is reportedly not being taken to making both of these issues the subjects of proper epidemiological studies on the widest possible basis.

Finally, the geographical approach or medical geography analytical epidemiological tool is a new venture that would prove quite relevant to both the ecology of Hansen's disease and the pattern of health care delivery systems, as proposed by Brightmer (1989) in the light of her experience in Nigeria, in that "the geographical approach in analysis begins by mapping prevalence and incidence rates of disease, and examining possible relationship with distribution patterns of environmental and/or socioeconomic features."

- At the level of medical care, it would be a truism to speak of irregularity of treatment in Hansen's disease. Much more serious is the fact that treatment is available for only one patient in five or four in a context of an estimated 12–15 million, of whom about five million are registered, 82% of these registered cases being from six countries (Zuniga, 1988). As regards multi-drug regimen (MDT), ever since its introduction in 1982, only 1.3 million patients benefit from it (Noordeen, 1984), a figure admittedly increased by now. Yet, the remaining three million-plus patients have to do with dapsone alone.

As regards the large failure attributed to patient treatment compliance, or non-compliance, it represents a significant, if not major, factor in the control of Hansen's disease. In this respect, the patient's behavior, as remarked by Georgiev and McDougall (1988), is influenced by a "complex mix of cultural, sociological and psychological factors, including his own beliefs as to what is effective treatment."

In her study dealing with the causes and related psycho-social dimensions of the phenomenon of non-compliance, Anandaraj (1986) looked at drug defaulting as a reflection of the underlying emotional, social, and cultural resistance elicited by the author,[3] striking a universal chord, she hypothesized—at least in her area— that the higher the awareness of Hansen's disease and the stronger the economic stability, the greater the motivation to be cured, other cognitive factors like caste, age, social standing, and educational status coming into it, too.

Whatever the other causes submitted and/or cognitive factors influencing non-compliance,[4] both equally important, there is, in the view of Vadher (1986), a lack of explanatory models of compliance, let alone single or simple explanation for non-compliance also.

Is not the patient more apt to cooperate if the modalities and rationale of this treatment be made explicit so as to impart sense to him? Levenstein (1988) goes further: "the issue that concerns us is not the merely narrow matter of compliance, but concern for the patient as a whole-concern respect, and attempt to understand the patient's world as reflected in the treatment situation."

Education of local medical practioners, on the whole poorly attuned to the existence of the disease in their areas, is unfortunately matched by insufficient training of paramedical personnel or peripheral health workers we are told, hence its direct bearing on the quality of medical care (viz. ready diagnosis or recognition of the first signs of the disease, follow-up or surveillance, reaching out for the patients, coping in time with immunologically-mediated reactions, disability and/or deformity, proper recording, etc.).

Poor patient compliance stemming from causes already elaborated—to which one should add inadequate instruction and lack of encouragement or guidance from medical and paramedical staff alike—is another bane of the control of Hansen's disease. Insufficient laboratory facilities on the whole and limited facilities for the ready referral of immunogically-medicated complications or reactions of the disease come into it, too.

Even though possibilities of reinfection await full investigations, there is besides the presence of microbial persistence, the high rates of primary dapsone resistance (in previous untreated patients) arising more quickly in some areas against a background for widespread secondary resistance (following dapsone therapy), quite a disturbing picture and cause for grave concern in respect of those countries (a reported 60%) not being able to afford multi-drug regimen.

The popular representation of Hansen's disease—traditionally thought of as the domain of voluntary agents and philanthropic organizations—is still linked to deformity when, as it has been seen, deformity is not attributable to the disease only. More dramatically, it has been estimated that some three million hansenians (leprosy patients) face the threat of permanent, progressive disability and/or deformity with its concomitant social stigmatization.

- Too much emphasis has been laid on the somatic aspects of the disease, too little on the equally important social and psychological aspects thereof, as has been made evident in this monograph. In other words, (i) not enough attention is paid to those aspects in the planning of control programs, (ii) firsthand knowledge of the prevalent attitudes of the community to the disease and the patient is lacking, (iii) both of which occur through an acute shortage of social workers as such, and of social scientists (viz. medical anthropologists, social psychologists, ethnologists, historians, medical geographers, etc.). This is illustrated by the extent to which social rehabilitation is lagging behind physical rehabilitation, as has been pointed out. It means that what is needed in the first place is a global study in endemic areas as regards the critical role of environment and behavior in the prevention of a disease like Hansen's disease, as has been recommended. The remark of Salins (1988) proves a familiar echo when she writes that:

The progress of leprosy control in large parts of the world is slow since the social aspects of the problem are not yet equally and effectively tackled along with medical treatment. A well planned extensive organized effort towards local rehabilitation of physical, economical, social as well as psychological aspects, is absolutely necessary.

Antia (1982) reminds us that the perpetuation of Hansen's disease as a major health problem or hazard is partly brought about by the "techno-bureaucratic approach having failed to understand or has ignored the significance of stigma which plays a predominant role in the disease without which appreciation no program for leprosy control can ever succeed."

In this context, let it be added that fear of the disease being as old as the disease itself, little wonder that in some endemic areas, even though they have access to adequate health centers, many hansenians (leprosy patients) shun treatment from fear of immediate social repercussions they know only too well, as has been reported. For Brand (1982), the most serious and stigmatizing complication of Hansen's disease is the belief by equally many patients that their condition is inevitably progressive, hence the futility or anticipated failure of treatment. Either way, (i) the patient's own set of beliefs, (ii) social stigma attached to the disease, (iii) the persistent fear of the disease, (iv) lack of community awareness and/or commitment, are not conducive to proper control of the disease too.

The principles of the much needed self-reliance on the part of the hansenians (leprosy patients) in view of avoiding dependencies of all sorts, however well promoted, fall short according to Godal (1978), of their goal through the human factor primarily involved. It means that a considerable length of time is still required for reaching a corresponding level of awareness to that effect.

In the meantime, as suggested by Huland (1988), it would be highly appropriate if the patients were motivated and/or trained as learners, i.e, what they need is learning about their condition, the price for neglect, and so forth.

As outlined so far, the overall picture—varying, admittedly, from region to region in both nature and degree—suggests that the day Hansen's disease will be relegated to the annals of eradication has not dawned yet, a forcible enough reminder of what ought to be done about it still. In other words, the fate of the disease—mostly under field conditions—is more than ever tied up with the need for cohesive policy and concerted determination at all levels since, as observed by Lechat (1981), medical means alone will not solve the problem.

However, new perspectives in terms of remedial measures are in the offing. With epidemiological tools like immunodiagnosis and immunoprophy laxis at hand, one would find out who is getting the disease, and by what mechanisms, or find out why some exposed individuals get it and others, equally exposed to it, not at all. In short, those epidemiological tools once made available would mean proper immunological intervention—as has been seen—i.e., primary prevention of the disease by stopping transmission at the source.

Epidemiological and operational research are promising in their activities, a multifaceted ongoing process implying (i) critical assessment of the validity and practicability of current indicators (viz. skin testing and serological techniques); (ii) establishing the portal(s) of entry of Hansen's bacillus (*M. leprae*); (iii) determining the interval between infection and onset of clinical signs; (iv) working out the epidemiology of disability and/or deformity; (v) probing drug resistance; and (vi) ascertaining the causes of relapse and or reinfection, as has been altogether described.

Of more immediate concern is the concept of primary health care (PHC) applicable to the control of Hansen's disease as well, another promising element fitting into present times which, like medicine, are changing.

The Central Variable

> Once operationally sound, primary health care (PHC) could well prove a major vehicle for controlling Hansen's disease, too.[5]

Health care delivery systems are, to a substantial extent, specific or relevant to local traditions, culture, resources, requirements, politics, and religion, as has been expressed, these, moreover, being co-critical determinants for health research strategy at the highest levels. In fact, as intimated by McKeon (1986):

> What needs to be done rather than the means by which it can be done . . . Large in concepts, clear in objectives and flexible in operation.

should serve as main guidelines to all those concerned with, or committed to the control of Hansen's disease.

At any rate, the general background to health care—particularly in Third World countries where it is dominated still by infectious disease—calls, once more, for a realistic outlook from the outset. Thus in the words of Bukman (1989):

> I am afraid that the outlook for many countries is gloomy. Many of them are faced with serious financial difficulties, notably the poorest countries with the fewest reserves, such as sub-Saharan Africa. Health care in these countries is hit by spending cuts stemming from structural adjustment programs. Indeed, in some countries health care has reached a crisis. This situation has produced a difficult dilemma: the need for adjustment is clear, but the need to maintain the present level of health care is no less obvious. I take the view that it is vital for humanitarian reasons to ensure that the radical changes which adjustment programs may cause are accompanied by measures to preserve essential educational and health care provision.

And again:

> If equity and essential health care are to be put into practice, the existing health service must undergo far-reaching restructuring. In practice, equity implies both a considerable increase in the number of

places where care is provided and the decentralization of the system. The introduction of equity is paralleled by the idea that care should be more effective to combat infectious disease from a large number of small-scale health care facilities than from a few large medical centers. These two principles likewise apply to the campaign against leprosy.

Community involvement being a key for the development of health infrastructures and the organization of health systems based on primary health care (PHC) units, it is equally well to take into account that:

Even though the general concept of community involvement has gained widespread support, there is little agreement on what the term means and little practical understanding of how it can be achieved. Therefore, it is essential to clarify what is expected for lay participation in health, including self-care, family "cover care," forms of indigenous social care-giving institutions, new social forms of health care, new social movements, structures for citizen and patient participation and new forms of legislation affecting health consumerism.[1]

Moreover, it is in the same context as well to remember that:

The human species is intensely social. This fact is so much a part of daily life that it is easy to overlook its significance. People everywhere are organized in societies. They repeatedly must choose between serving individual interests and those of the group.

And again:

Many of the developing nations are undergoing rapid social changes. These changes are having important effects on physical and mental health. They involve urbanization, industrialization, and large-scale migration as well as prolongation of uncertainty about adult roles, unemployment, vast increase in scale of the community of reference, and greater cultural heterogeneity.
Taken together, these factors tend to weaken and even rupture the fabric of traditional cultures and attenuate their socializing, orienting and supportive functions. This weakening of traditional family and community roles may have a critical impact on health-relevant be- havior, especially when the vital social functions are not supplanted in other ways.[1]

The above preambles are meant as prerequisites to one's appreciation of the concept of primary health care called upon to play eventually a major role in the control of Hansen's disease, too. More than a resurgence over the past decades, rather the extension of community development movement instead, primary health care presently enjoys a vogue within a universal climate of optimism, as has been remarked. Basically, it implies breadth as opposed to depth, i.e., a "horizontal" approach to health care delivery systems, with a view to replace—or phase out—the sophisticated, target-oriented, "vertical" approach thought in many quarters to be a significant factor of failure in disease control. A major reason for this is that the "vertical" approach proved to be neither technically nor economically paying off on a large scale, nor feasible and acceptable politically and psychologically, as has been explained.

What is fundamental to the concept of primary health care is that the patient, in the words of J.H. Levenstein (1988), is considered "whole rather than an ever diminishing fragment . . . not a number or a case or disease entity who fits into one or another category, but a whole person, the meaning of his disease acknowledged as being unique to him, or her." In the view of the author, another major aspect of primary health care is "recognizing the relationship between doctor and patient, patient and family with environment through a trusting, ongoing relationship, and universally accepted as such." As regards primary health care itself, Levenstein has three more important points:

(i) PHC is not a vocation, but an autonomous, non-differentiated or holistic discipline on the interface between society and traditional specialized medicine bent on tertiary health care and its potential sequelae, namely depersonalization of the patient; (ii) the very essence of PHC is the personal, comprehensive and continuing care of the patient within two major areas of human commitments, namely prevention of disease and management of the chronicity of the disease; (iii) anything else would be second rate, and doomed to failure because it would have failed to take into account the individual sick patient.

What is more, "unless there is a sound primary level of health care, the rest of the system will be wasted, expensive and inefficient, no matter how skilled or how expert or how highly specialized it is."[6]

However much one does subscribe to the above, one ought, by the same token, reckon with the prevailing sovereignty of the medical establishment bent on tertiary practice and based on the principles of specialization and fragmentation, vested interests, the demands of society, health policy makers, and politicians at the expense of PHC.[7]

Granted that PHC is not an enterprise but community-oriented and community-based health care guided by the principles of self-reliance, i.e., the active participation of that community through the identification of its felt needs as remarked by Bijleveld (1982), it is well to remember that the community as the hub of PHC system is not monolithic by vocation: it varies from culture to culture with its traditional belief systems, its own set of customs and habits, standards and expectations, requirements and priorities, as is well known.

Another aspect worthy of consideration is that rural societies are, more often than not, strewn with conflicting interests, internal strife, or political factionalism of one kind or other, hence fragmented, as intimated equally by Bijleveld (1982). It would seem, then, that behind this sort of facade, from a public health view-point, the response to preventive measures as such does not usually meet with expected results, in that most rural people are more keen on the extent and quality of curative cure, equating that cure with the "magic" of the injection as opposed to the discipline of pill intake, a familiar enough episode for those with experience in the field.

However desirable the democratization of Hansen's disease, namely its insertion into the PHC delivery system as opposed to mass campaign on its own, it is to be borne in mind that rural people tend to consider the disease more as a public health menace than another communicable disease, hence they would prefer to having patients treated elsewhere, i.e., not at a primary but a secondary, even tertiary level, as has been pointed out.

The attitudes or set mentality of the community towards disease and patient as is the case with Hansen's disease ought to be taken more substantially into account, in fact "must never be underestimated if only because deeply held beliefs may rub contrary to received medical opinion and thus hamper control," as Cullinan (1982) puts it. In other words, deeply embedded local consciousness, attitudes, or set mentality referred to, are borne out not so much by the presence of the individual hansenian (leprosy patient) with or without deformities, rather by the stereotype he represents through the distorting lenses of the community members: to put it mildly, the archetypal outsider, as intimated by the present writer.

The concept of PHC is a pure product of Western approach to health care delivery system, thus while one takes for granted that one's medical training is First-World–oriented, do one's standards find that much favor among Third World populations? Does it even cross one's scientifically educated and/or "developed" mind that not addressing the needs and expectations of Third World patients in general might partially be a prime cause of the situation, i.e., in ways and means suitable to their understanding and cooperation? Does not one need to appreciate, in this case, the hansenian's (leprosy patient's) concept of his illness by understanding first the context with which that concept arises through his culture, beliefs and values?[8]

For instance, Africans in general attribute illness and disease either to a human agent, an inanimate object, or the supernatural, while his material circumstances are contributory factors.[9] Or, as Kaufmann et al. (1986) stated: "In African societies, it is generally thought that leprosy has a natural and supernatural cause, an important distinction because a disease which has a supernatural cause is considered far more serious than having a natural case." Moreover, those people, without access to appropriate sources of knowledge, have their own alternate or atavistic response through the power of traditional healers or medicine men, herbalists, diviners, faith healers or shamans, casters of evil spirits, as has been time and again pointed out.

With the above altogether in mind, it would be pertinent to ascertain the present degree of success of primary health care (PHC) in Third World countries and, by the same token, how many PHC units have already teamed up with the control of Hansen's disease worldwide, a disease notorious for "its difficult constraints and complications relating to its diagnosis, treatment and management," as defined by McDougall (1982). It would seem that the first has been a controversial issue since its inception; on the second count, reported successes are few.

Some authors like Ross (1982) believe that PHC "could be the greatest thing ever to happen for the cause of leprosy control— provided the leprosy health professionals grasp the opportunity being presented," and Buchmann (1982) saw in PHC the "most single promising solution to the control of leprosy in terms of an alliance based on a total worldwide health care approach."

Yet it would appear that the role of PHC in the control of Hansen's disease spells a cautionary tale, too, in that, as intimated by Cullinan (1982), a PHC delivery system that is appropriate in one country, or even in one area, may be entirely inappropriate in another. Bijleveld (1982) goes further into saying that the "reality of the field situation . . . suggests, however, that for the present it would be premature and counterproductive to divert effort or resources to this new approach (i.e., PHC). When and where a PHC project has managed to take root in the community and has, for many years, demonstrated that it is functioning effectively, the time will be ripe to introduce leprosy control into the project."

In short, while evidence that PHC meets the criteria for the control of Hansen's disease is wanting,[10] one is in agreement with Lechat (1985) that, before everything else, the moot point is "how to provide a workable interface between the community and the patients, the patients and health personnel."

The Promising Tools

> Primary epidemiological intervention or prevention, and not secondary prevention, is the key to successful control of Hansen's disease.

So far, secondary preventive measures or secondary prevention strategy—confined to case-finding, chemotherapy, follow-up, and health education based on clinical disease mostly—are the rule, yet thwarted by operational and technological limitations, with the result that the prevalence and incidence of Hansen's disease cannot be attenuated with reasonable periods of time, as has been submitted.

What is really needed are sero-epidemiological tools aiming at primary prevention, i.e., with a view to stopping transmission of the disease from man to man, the human host seemingly the only source of infection, as already intimated by Bloom (1985), and subsequently by Kaldany and Nurlign (1986). These tools, immunodiagnostic and immunoprophylactic in nature, are fortunately given top priority under the aegis of WHO.

Immunodiagnosis is essential for the detection of sub-clinical infection, or early diagnosis of the disease, as well as the early identification of high-risk groups of people. To this effect, apart from promising results obtained among healthy contacts of multibacillary and paucibacillary patients, Bharadwaj et al. (1989) find that the Fluorescent Leprosy Antibody Absorption Test (FLA-ABS) proves to be a highly sensitive one, too, for detecting sub-clinical infection in Hansen's disease, particularly so in younger age groups.

Immunoprophylaxis calls for the protection of populations at risk by means of immunological conversion induced by appropriate vaccines suitable to Third World conditions. In this respect, Bloom (1985) queries whether, through the application of modern technology, it will be possible to develop vaccines for the prevention of Hansen's disease, and wonders:

> Why there is little awareness that prevention of a disease, and the research that may be required, can prove infinitely less costly than the expense of treating or suffering the human consequences of disease. It is always easier to seek funds for drugs to treat illnesses than it is for supporting research to develop vaccines that will perhaps prevent disease.

As has been expressed, advances in molecular biology and immunology and increasing knowledge of the chemistry of Hansen's bacillus (*M. leprae*) offer possibilities with the production of immunogenic material (viz. antigenic peptides and glycolipids, anti-antibodies, monoclonal antibodies, etc.) acting as antigens and eliciting immune responses and/or defining antigens relevant for the induction of protective immunity or mediation of pathological response, the overall aim being a suitable vaccine.

Nordeen (1985) puts in a word of caution, in that:

> It should be pointed out at this stage that no matter how promising are the newer tools such as vaccines, they do not automatically guarantee that leprosy control shall be achieved. Experience has shown that the problems in the application of even the most efficient tools for effective control are often more difficult to surmount than the problems in the development of the tools themselves. The implication is that leprosy

control programs should learn to use the existing tools such as modern chemotherapeutic regimens to the maximum effect through improved operational performance and be in a position to accept even better tools and apply them efficiently as and when they become available.

And subsequently (1988):

Leprosy poses some unique problems in relation to vaccine prospects. Firstly, we need to know more about sub-clinical infection in order to discriminate between the infected and uninfected in the non-disease population and evaluate the role of the vaccine in the two groups. At present we do not have a tool, whether serological or skin test, specific enough to make this discrimination. Progress in IMMLEP indicates that such tools may become available in the near future. Secondly, with regard to the occurrence and pathogenesis of lepromatous leprosy and its immunological unresponsiveness, we do not know whether it represents a mechanism which can be interfered with through a vaccine to the advantage of the infected person. Thirdly, there is apprehension that immulogical upgrading of the population through the vaccine may result in an increased occurrence of tuberculoid leprosy at least in the initial period following vaccination.
Lastly, we do not know enough about the role of mycobacteria and "M. tuberculosis" in influencing the epidemiology of leprosy and how they might interfere with the efficacy of the vaccine one way or the other.

Some authors like McDougall and Yamalkar (1987) feel that owing to the long incubation period of Hansen's disease, the vaccinated populations will have to be observed for at least ten years before the protective action of a vaccine against the disease can be proved. Other authors have expressed their doubts that, if proven, the role of immunogenetics in Hansen's disease might have no salutary effect on the development of the polar multibaccillary (PM) or LL form of the disease. Others, still, acknowledge the disease would be, indeed, the best hope for Third World countries where a vaccine against the disease is endemic, provided, though, that it be (i) inexpensive, (ii) readily available, (iii) easily distributed in a non-frozen form, (iv) administered with a needle not needing sterile conditions, and (v) safe or with minimal side effects.

The Vital Link

> The reported lack of conspicuous success of health education in Hansen's disease underlies the necessity of dealing with the problem of stigma in the first place.

It would seem that, in matters of health, "teaching people to know what they ought to know is just as important as teaching them to behave when they do not behave," two prerequisites that do not always fit into the strict observance of live facts. While programs in health education abound as much in their diversity as their unfailing theories, guidelines, and recommendations, what is at issue is the worldwide evidence that health education in Hansen's disease is not yielding the expected results, a matter subject to revision for many, a cause for concern for some, a failure for others.

Critical appraisal of the various approaches to health education in Hansen's disease falls outside the pale of this monograph, yet it is the contention of its author that principles of health education pertaining to that disease are valid as long as: (i) relevant, meaningful and applicable to the realities of the disease on a community basis; (ii) consistent with local culture in terms of current beliefs, practice and attitudes of the people concerned; (iii) fostering educational skills in respect of both health worker and patients alike; (iv) making use of specialized communication methodology in the vernacular; (v) taking advantage of mass media expertise; and (vi) achieving, in the final analysis, a stepwise yet genuine change of health behavior in people of endemic areas particularly.

However time-consuming, producing behavior changes in the community towards Hansen's disease and the patient is the overall purpose, which stands a better chance of success through behavioral sciences, a case in point being the encouraging results obtained by Matthews et al. (1980) in India, namely through information, motivation, and action.

Yet one is reminded that the live fact, or the root and bark, of Hansen's disease from a psycho-social standpoint remains stigma, the import of which has been discussed previously in the text. It is felt that unless stigma is addressed in the first place and removed, it would most likely mean further avoidance of detection of the disease until it has developed into a more advanced stage, hence making more difficult the prospects for treatment and cure as has been observed, not to mention further social ostracism for the hansenians (leprosy patients). Antia (1982) brings the point home when he writes that:

> Should we not then try to study the real causes of stigma as it affects the various segments of our population and how they perceive the disease and its sufferers? Should we not find out why the medical profession itself has such an unscientific fear of the disease as it has of no others? Can we expect health education to succeed when the medical profession which is looked to for guidance on medical problems refuse to handle leprosy patients and admit them to hospitals? In actual fact, stigma is most marked in the educated and not so great among less educated masses. Yet being the decision makers, whether in medicine or employment, they play a major negative. role . . . A better understanding and appreciation of the human aspects of this disease is essential in devising any program for its control, the lack of which has been the major cause of our failure.

However complex the nature of stigma, there is neither disregarding nor denying (i) its disastrous effects on the hansenian (leprosy patient), as well as a major impediment to both health education and control of the disease; (ii) hence the urgent need to develop an overall strategy for its eventual removal, an endeavor less formidable if undertaken stepwise and systematically by:

- Finding out the true nature and extent of stigma in endemic and partially endemic areas, notwithstanding its long-term psychological and social repercussions that persist after successful therapy; and
- devising ways and means to depolarize or defuse the nefarious consequences of stigma, by (i) fighting it on its own ground through the "wisdom of putting a face to it," as has been already suggested, and (ii) removing the very label "leprosy" which, as has been similarly said, anticipates and recapitulates stigma; thereby paving the way to a more fruitful health education in favor of Hansen's disease.

The Cinderella Discipline

It is crucial for the strategy of rehabilitation to ensure a high degree of community involvement, as well as the active participation of both the patient and his family.

Rehabilitation fits into the continuum of health care responsibility and the control of Hansen's disease, both of which embody traditional yet similar levels of prevention, i.e, tertiary prevention or the Cinderella discipline, a term used by Disler et al. (1984) yet not devoid of contentious issues. For instance, the authors wondered whether limited resources should be expended on the rehabilitation of the disabled people for an already overflowing labor market and/or in the light of the increasing unemployment rate in Third World countries, or whether one could really rehabilitate a person who comes from a serious disadvantageous socioeconomic background.

Such considerations fall outside the ken of this monograph, its author, moreover, subscribing to the view that rehabilitation of the hansenian (leprosy patient) in his identity and integrity is an imperative for all those concerned directly and indirectly with Hansen's disease. As Brand (1988) puts it:

> Any leprosy program which fails to address the patients' disability and dislocation from society, is, especially from this perspective, a failure.

And again:

> Rehabilitation is not an additional service to leprosy control, that can be left out if funds are limited. It is fundamental to the success of control, which may be waste of money without it.

Tradition has it that, so far, rehabilitation of the hansenian (leprosy patient) in both endemic and non-endemic countries is left to the humanitarian care and specialization of voluntary agencies and philanthropic organizations, yet mainly on an institutional basis. Whereas there is little doubt that a lot of good work and dedication is going into it, and that it is heartening to hear of the promotion of specific measures and the advocacy of more effective approaches and technologies from some governments, as has been reported, it would seem that, on the other hand, (i) motivation at different levels, (ii) utilization of available resources, and (iii) staffing and training for the purpose are not altogether commensurate with the needs and magnitude of the problem.

Ideally, rehabilitation should be envisaged upon the first signs of neural impairment, and initiated by means of appropriate measures that would eventually ensure the restoration of the hansenian (leprosy patient) to the fullest possible mental, emotional, vocational, and economic usefulness of which he is capable, as has been emphasized.

In reality, this sort of restoration is confined to a fairly restricted number of patients in the endemic and non-endemic areas, and under particular conditions. In practice, it is hardly the case on a government-sponsored national basis. By and large the unwarranted fear and/or unjustified revulsion of the handicap patient is looming over the whole issue of rehabilitation with its trail of latent opprobrium.

Admittedly, not all hansenians (leprosy patients) are amenable to rehabilitation, and each and every one of them is to be selected and/or treated on his own merit, as has been submitted. Human nature going its unpredictable way, it is hardly surprising to hear that a good proportion of handicapped patients prove unconcerned or indifferent, lazy or apathetic, resigned or fatalistic, unsettled or itinerant: many of them have chosen instead the more lucrative profession of beggars, as is well known.

Granted that there usually is a discrepancy between theory and practice, i.e., between policy and experience, power and decision, ruling and implementation, the point is how to rehabilitate the hansenians (leprosy patients) with medical, psychological, educational, and economic support to which they are entitled. Should it be on humanitarian grounds alone, when after curing the disease there is no guarantee that they shall be free of the yoke imposed on them? It would seem that the proposition depends on the first place on whether the patients become, or are made, personal enough for the rest of the community to accept them and their disease, and, by the same token, adopt fundamental changes in behavior.

Or, as Gill (1968) asks:

Then how are they (the patients) to be rehabilitated? What is meant by rehabilitation? Rehabilitation means to restore a person mentally, physically, economically, and socially into society so that he may become independent of outside help. Social, physical and economic and psychological stability are the pillars on which the temple of rehabilitation stands.

At this juncture, a brief review of some cognitive yet far reaching observations is deemed warranted:

- Health authorities are generally less concerned with an illness like Hansen's disease which, in their estimation, pales in significance when compared, for instance, to cancer, cardiovascular accidents, mental disorders, or AIDS, as has been intimated.
- What the public at large and society in particular think of the disease is, to an appreciable extent still, bound subconsciously to biblical, if not medieval, concepts.
- Hansen's disease does not as a rule attract or retain the attention and/or interest of the medical profession as such: as an illness set apart, it is left to those concerned directly or indirectly with it.
- Poverty, racial and minority status, tribal differences, caste system, and atavistic opprobrium remain alienating factors, in that they prove obstacles to rehabilitation.

It would seem that the issue of rehabilitation hinges on three prerequisites to be borne in mind: the hansenian (leprosy patient) himself, the community to which he belongs, and the responsible health authorities. Thus:

- It is evident that the hansenian (leprosy patient) ought at the onset to have enough will power and/or desire to undergo the full process of rehabilitation, or eventually be helped to help himself until satisfactory results be obtained. Alternatively, ways and means are to be found to talk him into it.
- It is generally acknowledged that in a community where Hansen's disease posits a health problem, tolerance on the part of that community is the exception, rather the rule, (i) thus inducing the patient to conceal the nature of his illness in its early treatable form as long as possible; (ii) hence, the attendant development of disability and/or deformity and (iii) the concomitant perpetuation of the endemicity of the disease in that area, as altogether observed by Browne (1981). It follows that to put up, from a com-

munity standpoint, a workable and lasting re-integration of the hansenians (leprosy patients) under the free label "rehabilitation" would mean (i) coming to grips with the psychological, social and cultural factors that determine the community's ingrained attitudes to both Hansen's disease and the patient; and (ii) dealing with people's thinking habits, cherished opinions, or traditional belief systems, with a view to increasing the awareness of those people by making them health conscious to the point of accepting the disease and the patient; in short, offering the hansenian (leprosy patient) an option within a context no longer nurtured but modified by those very factors.

While it is clear that unless the community modifies its relationship with both the disease and the patient—as has been repeatedly advocated elsewhere—through a due process of change, any attempt at rehabilitation would mean paying lip service to it, it would appear that the missing dimension is more than a sense of personally being sympathetic to the issue: rather, that sort of understanding beyond mere charity. In other words, the determination to help in breaking down the very barriers that make the hansenian (leprosy patient) still an outcast among the members of his community.

Individually, a feasible endeavor; collectively, seemingly an exercise in futility or an impossible task somehow left to the upcoming generation(s), in the hope that both disease and patient will be looked at with different eyes through a more compassionate yet meaningful attitude towards, equally, those in need of sustained help.

- Authorities dealing with health care delivery systems have their particular share of responsibility, in that the onus is on them for promoting and ensuring, in this case, rehabilitation of the patient in the fullest possible sense through community participation. Any other way would be doomed to failure by virtue of a commonly agreed-upon principle: the more restricted the area of operation, the greater the chance of implementing a given policy on a practical and sustained basis.

This is feasible through each available and functioning PHC unit under suitable guidance and proper supervision, or through community-based rehabilitation as opposed to institution-based rehabilitation costwise advocated by the WHO, hence ensuring a better chance of community awareness and involvement (Noordeen, 1984). Either way, it would prove a major step forward, the success of the scheme, though, remaining a function of the extent to which the fate of the hansenian (leprosy patient) would have been, in the meantime, truly alleviated.

Reverting to the remark of Antia (1982) concerning stigma, there is no doubt that its removal applies equally to the rehabilitation process: what is a major obstacle in the control of the disease is proving an impediment in rehabilitation, both within a similar context of popular ignorance, prejudice and fear. In the same vein, Rotberg (1979) reports that the implementation of the Third Phase of Prevention in Brazil is coping with both a national campaign of destigmatization whilst dealing concurrently with rehabilitation, yet with the reservation that what is suitable in Brazil might not be applicable elsewhere. Either way, it strikes a note of urgency at the heart of health care delivery systems whereby fighting what is called "leprostigma" would equally ease rehabilitation.

On both accounts, it implies a front-line strategy for filling in the gap between community awareness and involvement, self-reliance and responsibility, through an optimal utilization of economic resources, and the participation of all those concerned with control of Hansen's disease and rehabilitation. An ambitious enough strategy, no doubt, but one that, while focusing on the hansenian (leprosy patient) as a person to be, by the same token, restored in his identity and integrity, would enhance, or even enlighten, the much needed change in attitudes from the public at large and society in particular, let alone from lay and professional upper echelons.

The hope of the present writer lies in that direction.

Notes

1. WHO Advisory Committee on Health Research Strategy (1986).
2. It is well known that the lower the prevalence of Hansen's disease in an area, the less the awareness of the disease, the less likely the chance of the latter to be suspected. In other words, in areas of low endemicity, the "index of suspicion" mentioned by Wheate and Harris (1987) would be correspondingly absent, hence a lower experience and/or practice of the disease locally.
3. In order of frequency: not convinced of the validity of treatment; choice of other physicians (presently not being treated); no time; no belief in medicine; fed up,

not interested; treatment too long; clinics too far away; thinking that the disease is cured; neglected, fate; in-law interference; fear of being detected; other complications.
4. In general: lack of awareness and/or support from the community; lack of personal commitment and/or motivation by the infrastructure (health workers); failure to cope with the problem through inadequate instructions and guidance; unfavorable doctor-patient relationship. On the patient's side: stigma, illiteracy, ignorance and/or deficient knowledge of the disease's causation, transmission and duration; lack of awareness of the seriousness of the problem; escape mechanism; fear of being tagged "leper"; the new problem of primary and secondary drug resistance; deep-rooted beliefs and attitudes to the disease (viz. God's will, curse of God, fate, sin, heredity, sexual immorality, witchcraft, etc.).
5. Primary health care (PHC), as defined by the International Conference devoted to it in Alma-Ata, 1978, implies essentially: "Health care made universally accessible to individuals and families in the community by means acceptable to them, through their full participation and at a cost that the community and country can afford. It forms an integral part of both the country's health system of which it is the nucleus and the overall social and economic development of the community."
6. *Journal of the Academy of Family Practice/Primary Health Care,* Republic of South Africa (1988).
7. Let us not delude ourselves: high technology medicine and its increasing sophistication brings in its wake further isolation of the patient, emotionally or otherwise as has been pointed out. Tertiary medicine, entrenched within the medical establishment, maintains its time-honored grip on society at its political and economical best, as has equally been remarked. On the other hand, health priorities are in the hands of health administrators, medical engineers, and opinion molders, who, under the aegis of government agencies, haven't on the whole the foggiest idea of what is human pathology at both physical and psychological levels.
8. Namely exposure, deprivation, destitution, and unequal educational and economic opportunities and/or resources on the whole.
9. While these are essential in understanding human behavior, they are not intractable variables, in that they are manipulable (mostly in the poorest rural areas of Third World counties) whether by man or circumstances to the benefit or disadvantage of the community. In other words, of all the cognitive factors that influence health status of a community, culture, values, and customs would seem to play a secondary role, as has been advocated.
10. I.e., sound practical knowledge of the socioeconomic and psycho-social factors of the community, understanding and cooperation to the full by its members, employment of local health workers, supervision and guidance of the PHC staff, and effective referral system, as has been stressed. Browne (1981) is of the opinion that "The secret of primary health care success lies in the extremely careful selection, training and supervision of auxiliary staff," and that it would be a shortsighted policy to do otherwise.

References

Anandaraj, H. Psychological Dimension of Drug Default in Leprosy. *Ind. J. Lep.* 58(1986): 424–430.

Antia, N.H. Leprosy: Primary Health Care: The Mandwa Project. *India. Lep. Rev.* 53(1982) 205–209.

Bharadwaj, V.P. et al. Immuno-epidemiological Studies on Sub-clinical Infection in Leprosy. *Int. J. Lep.* 57(1989); Abstr. Cong. Pprs. FP 133: 329.

Bijleveld, I. In Reality: A Medical Anthropologist's Reservations About Viability of Leprosy Control Programs within Primary Health Care. *Lep. Rev.* 53(1982): 181–191.

Bloom, B.R. Towards a Leprosy Vaccine. *World Health* (May 1985): 3–5

Brand, M. Recommendations on Rehabilitation. Pre-congress Workshop. *Lep. Rev.* 59(1988): 284–307.

Brightmer, M.I. The Role of Geographer in Leprosy Research and Control: Case Study from Nigeria. *Int. J. Lep.* 57(1989); Abstr. Cong. Pprs. FP 098: 322.

Browne, S.G. Social and Vocational Rehabilitation of Leprosy Patients in Asia. ILO/DANIDA/Asian Regional Seminar, Bombay (1981): 3–7.

Buchmann, H. The Potential Benefit of Primary Health Care of Leprosy Control. *Lep. Rev.* 53(1982): 211–220.

Cullinan, T.P. Primary Health and Leprosy. *Lep. Rev.* 53(1982). 221–226.

Disler, P.B. et al. Whither Rehabilitation? Editorial. *S.A. Med. J.* 65(1984): 829–830.

Forster, R.L. et al. Nutrition in Leprosy: a Review. Editorials. *Int. J. Lep.* 56(1980): 66–81.

Georgiev, G.D. and McDougall, A.C. Blister Calendar Packs—Potential for Improvement in the Supply and Utilization of Multiple Drug Therapy in Leprosy Control Programs. Editorials. *Int. J. Lep.* 56(1988): 603–610.

Gill, I.K. Social Problems of Leprosy Patients. *Int. J. Lpr.* 36(1968); Abstrc. Cong. Ppr. XIII 157: 634.

Godal, T. The Clayton Memorial Lecture 1978: "Is Immunoprophylaxis in Leprosy Feasible? *Lep. Rev.* 49(1978): 305–317.

Huland, J. The Patient as Learner. *Int. J. Lpr.* 56(1988): 400; Abstr. Cong. Pprs. PO 528.

Kaldany, R.J. and Nurglin, A. Development of a Dot-ELISA for Detection of Leprosy Antigenuri under Field Conditions. *Lep. Rev.* 53(1986): 95–100.

Kaufmann, A. et al. The Social Dimension of Leprosy. ILEP. 3rd Ed., 1986.

Lechat, M.F. The Way Towards Eradication of Hansen's Disease. Sasakawa Memorial Health Foundation, 2nd. Ed., June, 1981.

Leiker, D.L. Opening Address, Europ. Lep. Conf., Genoa, 1981, Hlth. Coop. Pprs. 1(1982): 7–8.

Levenstein, J.H. Family Medicine, Medical Bureaucracies, and Society. *J.S. African Academy of Family Practice/Primary Health Care* 9(1988): 173–182.

Levenstein, S. Compliance—What's It All About? *S.A. Fam. Pract./PHC* (August 1988): 305–311.

Mathews, C.M.E. et al. Health Education in Leprosy. *Lep. Rev.* 51(1980): 167–171.

McDougall, A.C. and Yamalkar, S.J. Leprosy: Basic Information and Management. Ciba-Geigy, 1987.

McKeown, T. Health Research Strategy for Health for All by the Year 2000. WHO/RPD/ACHR 86: 13–20.

Noordeen, S.K. The Role of Rehabilitation in Leprosy Control. Int. Cong. on Rehab. of Leprosy Patient and Social Rehab. of the Disabled in Third World Countries. Rome, December 1984., Vaccination Against Leprosy: Recent Advances and Practical Implications. *Lep. Rev.* 56(1985): 1–3., The Present Status of Leprosy Vaccine Development. *S.E. Asian J. Trop. Med. & Pub.* Hlth. 19(1988): 525–534.

Ross, W.F. Leprosy and Primary Health Care. *Lep. Rev.* 53(1982): 210–204.

Rotberg, A. The Brazilian Phase III of Prevention of Hanseniasis. *Int. J. Derm.* 18(1979): 655–659.

Salins, S. Psychological Stress and Development of Leprosy. *Int. J. Lep.* 57(1989); Abstr. Cong. Pprs. PO 327: 361.

Shepard, C.. Leprosy Today. *New England J. Med.* 307(Dec 23, 1982), 26: 1640–1641.

Vadher, A. Factors Influencing Clinic Attendance for Treatment of Leprosy. *Int. J. Lep.* 57(1989); Abstr. Cong. Pprs. FP 228:348.

Wheate, H.W. and Harris, G.F. Operational Problems in Leprosy Control Programs when the Endemicity Declines. *Lep. Rev.* 58(1987): 1–5

WHO/RPD/ACHR (HRS): Health Research Strategy by the WHO Advisory Committee on Health Research, 1986.

Zuniga, M. Epidemiology. Pre-congress Workshop. *Lep. Rev.* 59(1988): 284–307.

Summing Up

> Much lies upstream, yet equally in keeping with the Hippocratic injunction that it is more important to know what sort of a person has a disease, than to know what sort of disease a person has.

In a little more than a decade those among us who will step into the twenty-first century are probably hoping to find in it, and beyond, the "New Millenium." They will seemingly be joining scientists and experts with a common purpose: not to be actors but participants in the future. Others, conscious of the sways of the present as portents of tomorrow, find themselves in a world blessed with technical prowess but singularly deprived of corresponding social and moral equivalents, as has been altogether remarked.

Some, still, stick philosophically to the unpredictable nature of the future and are prepared, instead, for the inevitability of change, the tempo of which is likely to be exponential in many areas of human endeavors, and more.

In the meantime, one is soberly reminded that

> Disease is not an inescapable attribute of the human condition, except when determined at or soon after fertilization: it results essentially from unhealthy ways of life and can be prevented if those ways can be changed.[1]

Bringing the point further home, Bloom (1985) asks:

> Why is there a general lack of commitment to the concept of international cooperation in health? It is profoundly sad and humiliating for a chairman of the Steering Committee, after successfully recruiting good scientists into the field of leprosy research, to have to tell an increasing number of them that their proposals for research in leprosy have been approved with good priority at the scientific level, but that there are insufficient funds to support the research project. This at a time when

a single jet fighter costs more than the entire WHO Programme for Research and Training in six tropical diseases. Why do the developed countries not make a greater commitment to the present and future health needs of the people of the developing countries? I am equally perplexed as to why leaders in many developing countries do not place greater emphasis on the health of their people relative to other priorities.

In this respect, Hansen's disease—and the expected success of its control—fit equally into the staggering agenda of the next century, as one of the multifarious yet concrete topics to be dealt with more realistically, perhaps to the extent of having to somehow "rethink" the disease.

In this monograph, major considerations give cognitive evidence that:

- The dignity and integrity of the hansenian (leprosy patient) are central to an issue concerning us all.
- The designation "leprosy" is, at best, "a historical misnomer" (Lendrum, 1952); at worst, "the corruption of an abusive term, a humiliating stereotype" far from being deprived of its actuality.
- The alternative terminology used through the text does, by virtue of its feasibility, reinforce the advocacy of the name change.
- It is no longer possible to envisage Hansen's disease otherwise than through its immunological roots, in that the spectral nature of the disease displays a diversity of clinico-pathological features which, in essence, are determined by, or derived from, the host-dependent variation in immune status against Hansen's bacillus (*M. leprae*) and its antigens. Moreover, whatever one can achieve in writing about it is bound, sooner or later, to be reformulated in the light of new findings, or readapted to a more appropriate language within the framework of basic research.

  It follows that (i) proper teaching of Hansen's disease warrants sound immunological premises, and (ii) the very definition of the disease be accordingly revised.
- Neural in its inception, Hansen's disease assumes its true status when dealt with from cause (primarily as peripheral neuropathy) to effect (secondarily skin and certain other tissue involvement), and not the other way around as has been hitherto the case.

151

- Hansen's disease eludes control against a multifactorial background, the term eradication not written in its history yet. While multiple drug therapy (MDT) is at the moment a major chemotherapeutic tool in the fight against the disease, only a reported 40% of the endemic countries can afford it. However important and worthy such a therapy, and those to come, the key to the control of the disease resides in primary intervention or prevention, a control that could be greatly enhanced by the removal of stigma, and the gradual implementation of the name change.

At this juncture, it is fair to acknowledge that an amazing lot has been found out about Hansen's disease over the past two or three decades while, at the same time—and unavoidably so—a good deal remains unclear or imperfectly understood, incomplete or inconclusive still. It would thus be more to the point to ask what is not known in the first place about the disease, rather than be satisfied with what has been achieved so far. The missing pieces of the puzzle are:

- The true magnitude of the problem worldwide (viz. prevalence and incidence of the disease, pattern of disability and/or deformity).
- Mode of transmission of the disease.
- The determinants that would explain (i) the latency or long incubation period of the disease, (ii) sub-clinical infection, (iii) the identification, development, pattern, and transmission of the disease.
- What determines whether the infection will be contained or will develop towards either polar form of the disease, or what factors determine which form of responsiveness will develop.
- The reasons for the interindividual variability of the disease on clinical grounds.
- As regards Hansen's bacillus (*M. leprae*) itself: the possible influence of its portal of entry; the mechanism by which itself and/or its antigens escape from the Schwann cell (extracellular release); the source of its energy for survival and proliferation purposes; its infective load; the complete identification of its antigenic components; its full biochemical and metabolic processes, as well as its genetical and molecular properties; why it chooses non-defensive

cells, or protected sites, that cannot be activated by the immune system; its relatedness or divergence (variability) among other strains isolated in different parts of the world.

- In terms of immunology: how soon the immune response is set into motion following initial infection; the exact behavior of the Schwann cell in relation to the immune system; the influence of genetics in the various forms of the disease developing after infection; the full immunological events in Hansen's disease, namely all factors determining the immune status of the host, or those triggering the host response to the antigens of Hansen's bacillus (*M. leprae*); the true nature of the selective unresponsiveness in polar multibacillary (PM) or LL patients, including its time of origin and reversibility; the full role of the immune cells and their sub-populations or subsets, individually and in unison.

More than is the case elsewhere in health matter, the all-too-familiar human factor pervades management and control of Hansen's disease, as made increasingly evident by the remarks of Lechat (1985), in that:

> Most unfortunate examples of prejudice may be given by doctors and other health personnel who outright refuse, or show their reluctance, to treat leprosy patients. Disregard for the individual needs of the leprosy patients, attitudes of superiority, indifference, and inefficiency of the health personnel, are the surest ways to keep the patient away.

Does it equally mean that this behavior falling short of its goal is linked to the likelihood that we are not taking in the facts of Hansen's disease to see them whole? That the reality of the disease has not reached the central pulse of awareness of people or that, perhaps, we are not enough responsible party to the grit of human condition?

The fate of the disease does not rest with theoreticians or cognoscenti by way of their own brand of tokenism: it depends on all authorities concerned with enough vision, and both administrative and political clout. For those in the front line, the way lies ahead, as intimated by Browne (1984). There is little doubt in the mind of the present writer that it calls for a broader, novel if not sharper focus on a fascinating and most challenging disease. It points to a more meaningful yet multidisciplinary knowledge of what to do about it, as has been expressed. It requires a constant revision of one's notions while taking into account current theories, hypotheses, and new findings. It demands standardization of criteria and uniformity of terminology, as postulated by McDougall (1982). It necessitates more basic research in all areas concerned and, chiefly, the means to achieve it.

Meanwhile, it causes mixed feelings to hear from Hastings (1989) that:

> At no time has there been more brain power, more enthusiasm, and more resources applied to the unsolved problems of the leprosy sufferer. No doubt as laboratory-based leprosy research becomes more and more sophisticated, it appears to be further and further removed from the frequently humble surroundings of the leprosy patient.

Here lies the paradox: science is progressing in favor of the hansenian (leprosy patient) more and more isolated, however unwittingly so. Here, after all is said and done, lies another illustration that, despite his accomplishments,

> . . . Man, proud man
> Dress'd in a little brief authority,
> Most ignorant of what he's most assured,
> His glassy essence, like an angry ape,
> Plays such fantastic tricks before high heaven
> As make the angels weep.[2]

Notes

1. WHO Advisory Committee on Health Research (1986).
2. William Shakespeare (1564–1616), *Measure for Measure.*

References

Bloom, B.R. Towards a Leprosy Vaccine. *World Health* (May 1985).
Browne, S. G. Leprosy. Documenta Geigy, Acta Clinica, 1984.
Lechat, M.F. Control Program in Leprosy. In *Leprosy.* Ed. R.C. Hastings (Churchill Livingstone, 1985): 253–268.
Lendrum, F.C. Leprosy. Correspondence. *JAMA* 222 (January 19, 1952).

GENERAL BIBLIOGRAPHY

Antia, N.H. Leprosy Control by a People's Programme: A New Concept in Technology Transfer. Current Lit. *Int. J. Lep.* 56(1988): 342.

Band, A.H, et al. Mechanism of Phagocytosis of Mycobacteria in Schwann Cells and their Comparison with Macrophages. *Int. J. Lep.* 54(1986): 294–299.

Benjamin, W.W. Healing by the Fundamentals. *New England J. Med.* 34(1984):595–597.

Bharadwaj, V.P. Ultracytochemical Studies of Lysomal Function in the Macrophage of Human Leprosy (I). *Int. J. Lep.* 55(1987):328–332.

Binford, C.H. et al. Leprosy. *JAMA* 247 (April 23–30, 1982), 16:2283–81.

Brand, P.W. Insensitive Feet. *A Practical Handbook on Foot Problems in Leprosy.* Leprosy Mission (1986).

Brandsma, W. Basic Nerve Function Assessment in Leprosy. *Lep. Rev.* 52(1981):161–170.

Browne, S.G. Letter to the Editor. *Lep. Rev.* 52(1982):321–322.

Cochrane, R.G. Biblical Leprosy—A Suggested Interpretation. *Life of Faith* 80(Jan. 19, 1958): 725–726.

Cohn, Z. A. et al. The Role of Lymphokines in Cell-mediated Immunity. *Int. J. Lep.* 53(1985): 725–726.

Convit, J. et al. Immunotherapy and Immunoprophylaxis in Leprosy. *Lep. Rev.* (1984) Special Issue: 575–595.

Corcos, M.G. Editorial. *Int. J. Lep.* 56(1988): 106–109.

Engers, H.D. et al. The Contribution of IMMLEP to Recent Advances in Immunology and Molecular Biology of M. leprae. *Int. J. Lep.* 57(1989); Abstrc. Cong. Pprs. FP 114: 326.

Fine, P.E.M. Immunogenetics of Susceptibility to Leprosy, Tuberculosis. *Int. J. Lep.* 49(1981): 437–454.

Gill, H.K. and Godal, T. Deficiency of Cell-mediated Immunity in Leprosy. Authors' Summary. Current Lit. *Int. J. Lep.* 55(1987): 177.

Godal, T. The Clayton Memorial Lecture 1978: "Is Immunoprophylaxis in Leprosy Feasible?" *Lep. Rev.* 49(1978): 305–317.

Grange, J.M. Mycobacteria and Human Disease. Author's Preface. Book Review, *Int. J. Lep.* 56(1988): 479.

Hastings, R.C. The 1985 Journal—A Continuing Perspective. *Int. J. Lep.* 54(1986): 88–108., The 1986 Journal. *Int. J. Lep.* 55(1987): 140–156., The 1987 Journal. *Int. J. Lep.* 56(1988): 82–100.

Harboe, M. Significance of Antibody Studies in Leprosy and Experimental Models of the Disease. *Int. J. Lep.* 50(1982): 342–350.

Hewitt, B. et al. The Most Vicious Circle in the Third World—Disease Causes Poverty—and Poverty Causes Disease. *Newsweek* (Dec. 1st, 1986).

Immunology. The Upjohn Company, Kalamazoo, Michigan, 1983. Scope Publication.

Jaret, P. Our Immune System: the Wars Within. *Nat. Geogr. Mag.* (June 1986): 702–34.

Jaroff, K. et al. Stop that Germ. *Time* (May 23, 1988): 52–63.

Kaplan, G. and Cohn, Z.A. Regulation of Cell-mediated Immunity in Lepromatous Leprosy. *Lep. Rev.* 57(1986); Supp. 2: 199–202., The Immunobiology of Leprosy. Author's Summary, Current Lit. *Int. J. Lep.* 55(1987): 177–78.

Kirby, R. The Dilemma of the First World S.A. Doctor and the Third World Patient. *S.A. Family Practice* (July 1988): 279–282.

Kolk, A.H.J. et al. Use of Monoclonal Antibodies in the Identification of Mycobacterial Antigens. Prov. IV Europ. Symp. on Lep. Res., Genoa, Oct. 1986, Hlth. Coop. Pprs. 7(1988): 101–106.

Lechat, M. Epidemiology of Leprosy. Europ. Lep. Conf., Genoa, 1981, Hlth. Coop. Pprs. 1 (1982): 29–32.

Longley, B.J. et al. Lepromin Stimulates Interleukin-2 Production and Interleukin-2 Receptor Expression In Situ in Lepromatous Leprosy Patients. *Lep. Rev.* 57(1986): 184–190.

MacKenzie, D. Leprosy: the Beginning of the End. *New Scientist* (May 3, 1984): 30–33.

Mahadevan, P.R. Host–Parasite Interaction in Relation to Leprosy. *Int. J. Lep.* 57(1985): 239–257.

Massey, E.W. Leprosy: Biblical Opprobrium? *Southern Medical J.* 71(1978): 1294–95.

Matsubara, H. Immunological Analysis of Leprosy. Current Lit. *Int. J. Lep.* 56(1988):659.

McDougall, A.C. Factors Influencing the Quality of Service of Leprosy Patients. *Int. J. Lep.* 50(1982): 355–358.

Muhkerjee, R. and Anita, N.H. Host–Parasite Interrelationship between "M. Leprae" and Schwann Cells "in vitro." *Int. J. Lep.* 54(1986): 632–638.

Noordeen, S.K. and Lopez-Bravo, L. The World Leprosy Situation. Rapp. Trismet. Statist. Mond. 39(1986): 122–123.

Noordeen, S.K. Current Global Strategy for Leprosy Control. Proc. of the Inauguration of China Lep. Assoc., China Lep. Foundation, China Lep. Control & Res. Center, Guanzhen, PRC, Nov. 1985., the Role of Rehabilitation in Leprosy Control. Int. Congr. on Rehab. of the Disabled in Third World Countries, Rome, Dec. 1984.

Pedley, J.C. The Stigma of Leprosy in Four Countries. *Lep. Rev.* 43(1972): 94–95.

Pontificale Academiae Scientiarum: Working Group's Conclusions on the Immunology, Epidemiology and Social Aspects of Leprosy, Documenta, Vatican City, 1984.

Punikai'a, B.K. Hansen's Disease: The Stigma, the Fear, the Solution. Abstrc. XIIIth Int. Lep. Congr., Amsterdam, 1988, FP 250.

Rotberg, A. Name Changes Reflect Trends. *Int. J. Lep.* 50(1982): 117–118., Letter to the Editor. *Int. J. Lep.* 54(1986): 648–649., Letter to the Editor. *Asian J. Med.* 8(Sept. 1972), The Brazilian Phase III of Prevention of Hanseniasis. *Int. J. Derm.* 18(1979): 655–59., "Hanseniasis" as a Substitute for "Leprosy." *Int. J. Lep.* 36(1968): 633.

Sansarricq, H. Recent Changes in Leprosy Control. *Lep. Rev.* (1983), Special Issue: S7–S16.

Sehgal, V.N. and Srivastava, G. Indeterminate Leprosy: A Passing Phase in the Evolution of Leprosy. *Lep. Rev.* 58(1987): 291–299.

Skinsnes, O.K. Letter to the Editor. *Lep. Rev.* 44(1973): 94–95.

Thangaraj, R.H. and Yamalkar, S.J. Leprosy for Medical Practioners and Paramedical Workers. Ciba-Geogy, 1986.

Torriani, C. Psychological Barriers to Rehabilitation of Leprosy Patients: Social and

Vocational Rehabilitation of Leprosy Patients in Asia. ILO/DANIDA Asian Regional Seminar, Bombay 1984.

UNDP/World Bank/WHO: Special Programme for Research and Training in Trop. Dis. 6th Rprt, 8, Lep. (1979-82)., 7th Programme Rprt. 8(1983-84)., 8th Programme Rprt.: The First Ten Years, 1987.

Watson, J.M. Preventing Disability in Leprosy Patients. The Leprosy Mission International, London, 1986.

Wheate, H.W. and Harris, G.F. Operational Problems in Leprosy Programmes when the Endemicity Declines. *Lep. Rev.* 58(1987): 1–5.

WHO Tech. Series 716, Geneva, 1985: Epidemiology of Leprosy in Relation to Control. 654, Geneva: Peripheral Neuropathies, 1980.

Author Index

Abel, I., et al., 57
Anandaraj, A., 128
Antia, N.H., 21, 122, 130, 146, 147
————et al., 111

Balfour, Lord, 45
Barnes, P.F., et al., 59
Baruffa, G., 43
Bechelli, L.M., and Ruffino-Netto,
    A., 108
Becker, I., 43
Berhan, T.Y., 86
Bharadwaj, V.P., et al., 65, 138
Bijleveld, I., 143, 144
Bloom, B.R., 1, 7, 50, 126, 137, 138,
    150
————and Mehra, V., 50, 58, 60, 64,
    66, 68, 69, 72, 107, 112, 145,
    146, 150
Boddingius, J., 105, 106, 119
Boillot, F., 103
Brand, M., 43, 142
Brand, P.W., 11, 14, 109, 130
————and Fritschi, E.P., 104, 109, 116
Brandsma, T.J., 114
Brightmer, M.I., 127
Browne, S.G., 10, 42, 43, 98, 103, 144,
    147, 153
Bryceson, A.D.M., 14, 50, 55, 65, 66,
    81, 93, 98
————and Pfaltzgraff, R.E., 90, 100,
    116
Buber, Martin, 45
Buchmann, H., 124, 125, 136
Bukman, P., 132

Campos, F.J., et al., 42

Camus, Albert, 43
Chakravarti, M.R., and Vogel, F., 57
Cockrane, R., 44
Convit, J., 37
————et al., 60
Cullinan, T.P., 135, 137

D'Almeida, L., et al., 42
Danielssen and Boeck, 1, 119
Davey, T.F., 21, 42
Del Cerro, S.G., 11
Demenais, F., and Feingold, N., 54
Dhople, A.M., 97
Diniz, O., 43
Disler, P.B., et al., 142
Dogliotti, M., 33, 40, 43, 44
Draper, P., 64, 73

Ell, S.R., 10

Faget, G.H., 43
Feldman, W.H., 40, 43
Fergula, V., et al., 59, 60
Ffytche, T.J., 43
Fleming, S., 13
Fleury, R., and Bacchi, C.E., 83, 99
Flynn, P.E., and Harvey, H., 12, 42
Foster, R.L., et al., 126
Fried, C., 44

Georgiev, C.D., and MacDougall,
    A.C.M., 128
Gill, H.K., and Godal, T., 58
Gill, I.K., 22, 143
Godal, T., 52, 59, 64, 65, 87, 107, 124,
    130
Goihman-Yar, M., 64, 65, 83

Goldman, L., 43
Gramberg, K.P.C.A., 43
Grey, J., 44
Grynpas, J., 44
Gussow, Z., and Tracy, S., 16, 17

Haidar, A.A.M., 21
Hamilton, G.R., 98
Harboe, M., 49, 56, 59, 65, 66, 69, 77,
     80, 89, 97, 100
Haregewoin, A., 59, 98
Hastings, R.C., 9, 98, 99, 109, 154
Hemerijckx, F., 6, 44
Hiatt, H.H., 44
Hill-Smith, I., 119
Holborrow, J., and Lessof, M., 64
Huland, J., 131

Job, C.K., 74, 85, 105, 107, 108
Jopling, W.H., 35, 37, 86, 89, 90, 91,
     98, 99, 100

Kaldany, R.J., and Nurglin, A., 137
Kaplan, G., and Cohn, Z., 59
Kaplan, J., 6
Kato, L., 98
Kaufmann, A., et al., 12, 15, 22, 23,
     97, 136
Khanolkar, V.R., 98, 103, 105
Kikuchi, I., et al., 57
Kircheim, W.F., and Storrs, E.E., 72
Kriel, J., 27

Lagrange, P.H., and Hurtrel, B., 49,
     65, 87
Languillon, J., 10, 42, 98, 99, 100
Latapi, F., and Zamora, A.C., 100
Lechat, M.F., 8, 10, 14, 43, 49, 50, 110,
     126, 131, 137, 153
Leiker, D.L., 125, 126
Lendrum, F.C., 18, 35, 40, 43, 151
Letayf, S., 12, 43
Levenstein, J.H., 26, 134
Levenstein, S.H., 128
Levinsky, N.G., 26

Lichtwardt, H.A., 5, 43
Liu Tze-Chun, et al., 80
Longley, B.J., et al., 59
Lucio and Alvarez, 101

MacDougall, A.C.M., 136, 154
MacDougall, A.C.M., and Yamalkar,
     S.J., 1, 42, 98, 139
Machin, M., 98
MacKeown, T., 132
Mahadevan, P.R., 66
Maier, M., 55, 58, 60, 99
Mallac (de), M.J., 5, 45, 119
Mangiaterra, M., 43
Mathur, D., et al., 74
Matthews, C.M.E., et al., 140
Mechanic, D., 27
Mehra, V.L.H., et al., 57, 58
Meisels-Navon, L., 10, 17
Mitchison, N.A., 64, 65
Modlin, R.L., et al., 55
Mshana, R.N., et al., 107
Mshana, R.N., and Nilsen, R., 49, 50,
     57, 58, 96, 98
Munoz, F.U. and Storkan, M.A., 42

Naipaul, V.S., 44, 45
Narayanan, R.B., et al., 98, 99
Nath, I., 54, 58, 60, 64
Newell, K., 57, 98
Neylan, T.C., et al., 2
Noordeen, K., 9, 73, 74, 98, 128, 139,
     146

Oliveira, N.L.W., et al., 32
Ottenhof, T.H.M., and de Vries,
     R.R.P., 9, 50
Ottenhof, T.H.M., et al., 60

Pettit, J.H.S., 98
Pfaltzgraff, R.E., 93, 100
Pfaltzgraff, R.E., and Bryceson,
     A.D.M., 100

Quiroga, M.I., 43

Rabello, F.E., 43
Ramos, T., et al., 56
Rea, T.H., and Modlin, R.L., 84
Rees, R.J.W., 73, 98
Rees, R.J.W., and MacDougall,
    A.C.M., 74
Reich, C.V., 74
Ridley, D.S., 75, 80, 81, 84, 86, 87, 88,
    91, 92, 93, 96, 97, 98, 99, 100,
    101, 105
Ridley, D.S., and Job, C.K., 72, 81, 83,
    89, 94, 95, 98, 99, 103
Ridley, M.J., 87
Ridley, M.J., et al., 87, 104, 105
Rolston, M.A., and Chesteen, H.E., 2,
    15, 17, 43, 110
Rosen, F.S., et al., 51
Ross Innes, J., 43
Ross, W.F., 136
Rotberg, A., 19, 25, 33, 43, 56, 57, 64,
    98, 100, 146
Ryrie, G.A., 42
Salins, S., 130
Salk, Jonas, 120
Samuel, N.M., et al., 77
Sankalia, N.S., 22
Scollard, D.M., 96
Shanmuganandam, S., et al., 11
Shepard, C.C., 97, 127
Sheriff, S., et al., 60
Shetty, V.P., and Antia, H.H., 105

Skinsnes, O.K., 2, 10, 12, 15, 18, 19,
    20, 21, 22, 24, 33, 34, 35, 37, 42,
    43, 44
———and Elvove, R.N., 23, 25
Skinsnes Law, A., 17
Smith, W.C.S., et al., 104
Souza, A.R., 43
Steiner, George, 43
Stonner, G.L., 60, 72, 86
Strickland, N.H., 54, 59, 65, 66
Stringer, T.A., 19, 38
Strober, A., and McDevitt, H.O., 64
Swellengrebel, J.L., 43

Tas, J., 9, 18, 42
Terence, 45

Van den Enden, W., and de Vries,
    R.R.P., 50, 57, 58, 60, 66
Van Voorhis, W.C., et al., 85, 90
Vhader, A., 128

Warren, A.G., 17, 34, 109
Waters, M.F.R., 98
Watson, Lyall, 5
Wheate, H.W., and Harris, G.F., 146

Young, D.B., 73

Zhou, D., et al., 13
Zukav, Garry, 6
Zuniga, M., 127, 128